ALL MY
WORLDLY JOY

ALL MY WORLDLY JOY

A Memoir of Motherhood and Mental Health

Laura Richmond

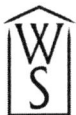

First published in 2025
Wilton Square Books
29 Wilton Square, London N1 3DW
www.wiltonsquarebooks.com
All rights reserved

© Laura Richmond, 2025

This book is a work of non-fiction based on the life, experiences, and recollections
of Laura Richmond. In some cases, names of people, places, dates, sequences
or the detail of events have been changed to protect the privacy of others. The author
has stated to the publishers that, except in such respects not affecting the substantial
accuracy of the work, the contents of this book are true.

While every effort has been made to trace the owners of copyright
material reproduced herein, the publisher would like to apologise for any
omissions and will be pleased to incorporate missing acknowledgements
in any further editions. Credits for quotations in copyright can be found on p. 312.

Typeset by Jouve (UK), Milton Keynes

A CIP record for this book is available from the British Library

ISBN 978-1-80677-013-7 (hardback)
ISBN 978-1-80677-012-0 (ebook)

Printed in Great Britain by CPI

1 3 5 7 9 8 6 4 2

Our authorised representative in the EU for product safety is:
Logos Europe, 9 rue Nicolas Poussin, 17000, La Rochelle, France
contact@logoseurope.eu

For Arthur, with all my love

With special thanks to Alain Gregoire at perinatalcourses.com, and Pirkko Koppinen

Contents

Notes on the Text

The events narrated in these pages are true as I remember them, but they are not the whole truth. Much has been omitted, and some names of individuals and locations have been changed. I've relied upon my own recollections, supplemented by letters, photographs, medical notes, and the diaries and notebooks I've kept since I was six years old. Memory is fallible, mine especially so, and, doubtless, mistakes will have crept in – these errors are mine and mine alone.

My observations are not grounded in any medical training but in my own experiences. I do not claim to speak for everyone.

I cover topics which may be distressing for some readers. These include descriptions of self-harm, eating disorders, birth trauma, mental ill-health, and psychiatric inpatient settings. Please take care of yourself while reading this book.

one

Bethany Fleamarket

It is an anxious, sometimes a dangerous thing to be a doll. Dolls cannot choose; they can only be chosen; they cannot 'do'; they can only be done by; children who do not understand this often do wrong things, and then the dolls are hurt and abused and lost; and when this happens dolls cannot speak, nor do anything except be hurt and abused and lost. If you have any dolls, you should remember that.

Rumer Godden, *The Dolls' House*[1]

Autumn 1996

Whenever you find yourself in possession of a large cardboard box, the best and only thing to do is to cut a hole in the front, climb inside, and pretend you're on television. Compose and perform your own adverts, complete with little jingles and snatches of song, for any objects lying around. Think of the most outrageous sequence of events you can and narrate it very seriously as if you were reading the news. Conclude every

3

broadcast with the following: 'How did it happen? Why did it happen?' – and in an ominous voice – 'Nobody knows.'*

I was fabulously wealthy when it came to large cardboard boxes. In the storeroom above the shop there was an endless supply of them, and of products to advertise. 'Soap on a rope!' I sang tunelessly. 'Where is the soap? It's on a rope! It's endorsed by the pope! Soap on a rope. Available downstairs on the bric-a-brac table. Terms and conditions apply.'

I was alone, a whole week of half-term stretching ahead. I could sit, unobserved and undisturbed, in my cardboard box and sing about soap on a rope in between bites of a Belgian bun the size of my head. I could wear my favourite dress. Like most of my clothes, this was handed down from older cousins. The skirt was bright orange with a yellow rickrack trim that billowed and flapped around my knees when I ran, and there was an orange hood to match. The bodice and sleeves were of a multicoloured geometric pattern, dominated by sludge green. The combined effect was magnificently hideous. It was a dress unlike other dresses, for a girl unlike other girls. I lived in it, completing the look with sandals, thick round spectacles that slid down my nose, and a halo of fluffy gingerish curls.

In the school holidays, I helped out – or, more accurately, hung out – at the shop. We always called it 'the shop' but its proper name was GJ's Fashions. It was owned by my uncle Bobby. *His* proper name was Graham but for some reason Dad always called him Nobby, or Norman. At some point I'd misheard or mispronounced Nobby as

---

* A favourite childhood game, heavily borrowed from an episode of *Rugrats*, an animated TV series on Nickelodeon.

Bobby, and so Uncle Bobby he was. Uncle Bobby was never at the shop; he was busy elsewhere. Mum said he was our answer to Del Boy off *Only Fools and Horses*. Dad was shop manager, which, when I was there, at least, meant popping in and out, and carrying boxes up and down the wooden stairs, while Nan sat at the till. I only ever saw Dad sit down when he was driving the big blue van around.

The shop stocked heavily shoulder-padded women's clothing: skirt suits in loud colours and velveteen gowns that pooled around my feet when I played dress-up. Most of what we actually sold was on the long table of bric-a-brac to one side of the shop floor. It was piled with soaps on ropes, boxes of novelty socks, porcelain clown ornaments, feather dusters, key rings with little fluffy chimpanzees in different colours . . . There was always plenty for me to play with, and there was the storeroom full of boxes upstairs and the changing room, where I could pull the curtain across to create a cosy little nook for myself. Nan sat in the corner beside the shop window, with the till which made a brilliant *WHOOSH-CLANG* noise as it shot out a drawer full of coins.

Ours was set in a row of shops beside Kingsland Market on St Mary Street, in a run-down inner-city district of Southampton. The area had a bad reputation, but I felt completely safe there. All by myself I ran errands to Biglands Bakery – a relic of a bygone era with its Art Deco shop front, *Bakers Confectioners Pastry Cooks* spelled out in stained glass above the door, and excellent Belgian buns – and to the Happy Shopper, and, of course, to the market itself.

The market had been there over a hundred years and

was once the city's prime shopping area. By the time I knew it, it was dwindling away and sold mostly fruit and veg, except on a Tuesday. Tuesday was fleamarket day, when the market roared back to life, and you could get just about anything: clothes, knitting wool, washing lines and pegs, toiletries, cleaning products, all kinds of meat, bricks of angel cake and madeira cake dotted with sticky glacé cherries, books, games, toys, and tat from dead people's houses. The last of these drew me like a magnet: fold-up tables stacked with a random assortment of miscellaneous objects from the previous few decades. Things in all their glorious thinginess, quite unlike our bric-a-brac, which was new. Nan would give me a couple of pounds to spend, and I'd wander around, breathing everything in – the noise, the bustle, the calling of the vendors – before finally allowing myself to settle reverently in front of this treasure.

St Mary Street was a disjointed array of buildings of different ages and designs, and it had a disjointed array of human beings within and around it. The market vendors, regular customers, and people who ran the shops along the street all seemed to know one another. They would arrive at the shop, removing hats and coats or shaking off umbrellas in the doorway, briefly cast an eye over our bric-a-brac table, and talk to Nan about everything and nothing for as much time as they could spare.

'Laura, my love!' Nan called across the shop and up the wooden stairs. 'Mrs Lilley is here!'

I extracted myself from my box and hurried to fetch Mrs Lilley a chair. I liked Mrs Lilley. I liked the way she talked not only to Nan but to me and to any dolls I had with me, and she took the time to learn and remember their names. I liked the pride in her voice when she spoke of her husband, an aeronautical scientist who had played a key role in the development of Concorde. Most of all, I liked hearing about the enormous collection of dolls she had at home. She had promised I could come to tea one day and see them all. I wasn't sure if this meant that I was actually going to her house for tea, or if it was one of those things that people say and don't mean, but since then, I had been especially attentive to Mrs Lilley.

'Such a good girl,' said Nan approvingly, as I dragged a chair across the shop floor.

My nan – or Nanny Bett, to give her full title – had an extraordinary gift for chat. She was warm and homely with friends and strangers alike. Reminiscence was her forte: she played the past like a musical instrument, and she had a shared history, it seemed, with the entire human race. With older people, like Mrs Lilley, she would talk about the war, and about a lost world where milk bottles were delivered by horse and cart; a world in which children played with wooden spinning tops, and sweets were kept in enormous glass jars labelled with intriguing names like humbug and barley sugar. It was a strange, distant, lovely world, softened by time, and they spoke of it with such feeling. They spoke as if it were just in the next room.

When the shop was empty, I had Nan all to myself, and she told me stories about her life. I knew them all by heart. How her father had left when she was three and she and her siblings were sent to the workhouse.* How one day

---

* What Nan always referred to as 'the workhouse' was actually a 'cottage home': a separate space established by some Poor Law authorities to house pauper children.

she wrote an essay which won a competition, and the prize was a year's supply of chocolate, but she had to share it with all the other children in the workhouse, which meant she hardly got any. How her schoolteacher was wicked and made fun of her in front of the class because she couldn't draw a daffodil. Years later, one of her sisters would tell me the unsanitised version of this childhood in the workhouse. I was appalled. Nan had always made it sound like the opening of a Roald Dahl book: cartoonish, not quite real, to be redeemed at any moment by magic that was just around the corner.

Then there were all the war stories. Nan had been conscripted at seventeen and ordered to report to barracks in Leicestershire. She'd never been on a train in her life and so she bribed her fourteen-year-old brother to come along and help her cross London. She left him at the barracks gates without a thought to how he would get home. From there she travelled all over Europe. Her official job, she said, was to look up at the sky and shout, 'Ready . . . aim . . . FIRE!' Her unofficial job seemed to have been chief practical joker of the Auxiliary Territorial Service.* Once, she had missed the drill – a sort of marching about every day for no reason – because she had to have her ears syringed. When she got back to the dormitory, they were all still marching, and she fiddled with the underside of her friend's camp bed so that when her friend got in and collapsed on the bed, exhausted, it snapped shut – (she always clapped at this point) – forming a sort of human

---

* The women's branch of the British Army during World War II. Queen Elizabeth II was also in the ATS, though I don't think Nan knew her personally. She would have mentioned that.

sandwich. She laughed whenever she recounted this as if remembering for the first time.

That was my Nanny Bett in her eighth decade – storyteller; soap-watcher; voracious reader of large-print Catherine Cookson novels; archivist of films taped off the telly and stored in VHS cases designed to resemble leather-bound books; singer of wartime hits and obscure folk songs; player of card games like Ha'penny on the King and Knock Your Neighbour Out of Doors; keeper of the little plastic bags full of 1p and 2p coins for gambling; and a prolific knitter who took custom requests. She was exactly what a nan should be. She took my side unequivocally and called me an angel unironically. She was also a very gifted hugger. She had a particular smell – a nice smell, musty-sweet. It was the smell of her make-up, thick beige-brown liquid foundation squeezed out of a tube.

In hindsight, I think we were so close partly because Mum had postnatal depression after I was born, and Nan stepped in to help, but also, we had the sort of family set-up that facilitates closeness. I had dozens of aunties and uncles and cousins, half of them on the doorstep. I couldn't walk the length of the high street without catching sight of three or four of my relatives. The family sprawled in the same way the city did, ever-expanding, overlapping, trip-ping over itself as it rumbled along the docks and out towards the countryside. You couldn't keep track of it, all veins and capillaries and one great, beating, maritime heart: a living, breathing support system.

My family were a tolerant bunch, mostly, and they allowed me to get on with being myself. Occasionally I overheard words like 'funny' or 'quirky', and even 'sensi-tive' and 'highly strung', but there was never any malice.

I had always known that there was something different about me. Something invisible. On the outside, I looked much like everyone else: two arms, two legs, nothing obviously amiss. But on the inside, something was different. I couldn't tell you what or why. It was just a feeling. Sometimes I noticed shifting glances and elongated pauses, and I knew that I made people uncomfortable. That made me uncomfortable. Somehow, I couldn't quite be myself when other people were around.

Still, when I was at home or with my family, it was all right. At home, different wasn't good or bad. It was just different. School was another matter. At school, different was bad. Different was wrong. I was starting to become terribly afraid that there was something wrong with me.

It wasn't the lessons. They were easy − too easy, in fact, like a class for babies. I was staggered at the apparent stupidity of my classmates, and I must have voiced this out loud because on at least one occasion I was pulled up for it and thoroughly told off. I was mortified, not just at the disapproval of my beloved class teacher but because I would never want to make someone feel stupid, even if objectively they were. Especially then. I understood how that felt, because there were things the others did − tie shoelaces, do handstands, swim, ride a bike − that somehow I could never manage. That felt horrible. But I seemed to have a knack for saying the wrong thing, however kind and friendly I meant to be. The children at school didn't like me, and those who did only liked me for a little while.

Playtime was like being a wounded gazelle in the African desert, a very loud, crowded desert with a lot of low-flying footballs. My classmates called me fat, because fat was the worst thing you could be if you were a girl. I was also a 'boffin' – someone considered to be unacceptably bookish or studious – and I was weird. That last one was fair enough: the more they hated me, the more I retreated into my own head and the more boisterously strange I became.

If you don't like the way things are and you can't change them, you can always imagine them otherwise and that's almost as good. It's wondrous, really; you can take yourself anywhere at any time. You can have your heart's desire for a spot of imagining. I found it helps to walk about: rhythm seems to aid the process. This led to a lot of wandering about the playground, or circling a particular tree, while involuntarily muttering to myself and gesticulating. That didn't exactly enhance my social standing. Nor did sitting with my coat over my head. If I'd had the confidence to embrace my strangeness and become a kind of kooky baby goth, I might have fared better, but I am, and always have been, deeply uncool.

Still, I liked being uncool in the school holidays. As I perched on the edge of Nan's chair beside the till, listening to her and Mrs Lilley, school was nothing more than a bad dream. When I was with Nan, different was good. Different was special. I was fully myself and I was fully happy.

—

I was on my way out of the Happy Shopper when I passed some lads doing 'penny for the guy'. They'd stuffed an old shirt and trousers and leaned them against the wall with a Halloween mask balanced on top, and a bucket to collect their earnings. They were big lads. Huge. Must have been at least fifteen, I thought. Their bucket was nearly empty, their expressions grim and restless. One rattled the bucket at me expectantly, nodding to the coins clutched in my fist.

I said, 'I've got to bring my nan the change,' and before I knew what was happening, these boys had grabbed me and prised Nan's change from between my chubby fingers. I ran away, howling.

Some kind soul returned me, still sobbing, to Nan at the shop. Nan called the police, and two policemen came. I had a ride in a police car. I was supposed to be spotting my assailants, but wisely they had made themselves scarce. By this time, I'd quite recovered and was thoroughly enjoying the attention. Word got around and people started dropping in – ostensibly to check on me, but also to hear all about it. Every time I told the story, it got a little more dramatic. By the fifth or sixth retelling, I'd almost been hurled through a shop window.

The first time I ventured out alone after my near-death experience, I went straight to the market. I couldn't miss the opportunity to go on a Tuesday. I plunged my hands, with the two £1 coins Nan had given me, deep into the pockets of my favourite dress and began to weave my way through the crowd. That was when I saw Bethany waiting for me on one of the stalls.

Bethany Fleamarket stood twelve inches tall, with fixed brown eyes and coarse, voluminous black hair. Her head was made of porcelain, as were her arms from elbow to fingertip and her legs from knee to toe. She wore a ruffled, old-timey dress, reminiscent of an Edwardian costume drama produced in the mid-eighties. She had a rigid stuffed body, which couldn't move or sit, sewn right up over her shoulder plate to her neck. She could only stare straight ahead, but it was clear to me that this tragic inflexibility of her body only enhanced the broadness of her mind. Bethany Fleamarket had worlds between her ears.

She had sound common sense and a knack for problem-solving. And she was very, very determined.

'You took your time,' said Bethany Fleamarket.

I approached the lady on the stall, who recognised me as the ringletted victim of a recent brutal mugging and gave me Bethany for nothing. Overjoyed, I spent my £2 on cake – it bought me quite a lot of cake – and took Bethany and my cake back to the shop. We sat on the floor of the changing room and pulled the curtain across.

'I wish people would attack me in the street every day,' I said cheerfully to Bethany, in between stuffing my face.

If the woman had given Bethany to me because she felt sorry for me or because she was kind, the real reason – the deeper reason – was that Bethany had wished her to do so. Doll-wishing, I mused, was a powerful force, one that was grossly underestimated in our notion of how the universe worked. Most events in human history, both tiny and momentous, probably occurred because, somewhere along the line, a doll had wished them into being. And Bethany Fleamarket was such an expert; she wished with such deftness, such precision, that she expended very little effort in causing a great many things to happen. She understood cause and effect.

She wished for a home for herself, where she would be suitably loved and venerated, and because she was a magnanimous creature, she wished the same for all dolls who languish at the back of dark cupboards. She wished that they would all find safety and they would find one another. She understood that I was exactly the sort of child to carry out this plan and would follow her instructions to the letter. When I got home, I arranged a sort of doll altar on the toy cupboard beside my bed.

Soon after, another porcelain doll waited and wished and waited on a fleamarket stall. Her name was One-Legged Margaret. Originally it was just Margaret, but one fateful afternoon I lifted her off the top of the cupboard by her hands and swung her over to the bed, chattering away. She fell in slow motion, hitting the cupboard door with a sound that was half smack and half crack, and lay in two pieces on the carpet. I cried. Margaret didn't cry, but only because she couldn't. Apologising endlessly, I wrapped the stump in sticking plasters, and she was One-Legged Margaret after that. There was always something rather tragic about her, even before she was One-Legged Margaret. Her blue eyes sparkled so that they always seemed brimful of tears, and she had Tipp-Ex on her face, where I'd tried to cover up some stray glue. Her knickers were held up with a safety pin.

And then there were three. Jane Hunt arrived, a gift from one of Nan's friends. Jane Hunt was a homemade rag doll with mismatched brown button eyes and woollen hair tucked under a bonnet. She was dressed in a soft pink calico print dress beneath an apron which had once been a net curtain. Her head was a bit floppy, so she had to be propped up carefully. I'd named her Jane Hunt after my favourite grave in the old 'boney' around St James' church:

IN MEMORY OF
JANE
DAUGHTER OF
WILLIAM AND ELIZABETH HUNT
WHO DEPARTED THIS LIFE
AUGUST 6TH 1862
AGED 14 YEARS
GONE BUT NOT LOST

I suppose most children don't have a favourite grave, but I loved that shady little churchyard near my school. I loved its ancient headstones, half legible, some mere stumps in the ground, and ivy spreading over everything like contagion. It was a peaceful place where I could roam the attic rooms of my mind, alone yet not alone. I had always felt more at home among the dead than among the living. Like dolls, their stories were malleable, their possibilities infinite, and there was something very safe about people who were half imaginary. I thought myself half imaginary too. I wasn't allowed to walk to and from school by myself, but I found opportunities to wander off unnoticed and visit the ghosts.

I'd even considered the possibility that I might be a ghost. What a plot twist that would be. It would explain why I was different from everyone else, why I felt such an affinity with the past and felt at home in cemeteries. I certainly never doubted that there were ghosts. On those rare and precious trips to the boney, I saw Jane Hunt as clearly as I saw anyone alive.

Did I believe that the ghost of Jane Hunt the girl came home with me in the body of Jane Hunt the doll? Probably. After all, she was gone but not lost. And it was exactly the sort of arrangement that Bethany Fleamarket would have orchestrated. Either way, Jane Hunt slept in my bed from the day that I named her. Once, I took her on a school residential trip and no one would take the bed next to me because they said she was creepy. Jane Hunt said she would rather be creepy than unkind.

These were the great triumvirate. I had other dolls too, loads of them – Barbies and Sindys, a singing mermaid, one with crimped hair which grew as you yanked her arm up and down, shelves full of those fancy display dolls on stands – but Bethany Fleamarket and One-Legged Margaret and Jane Hunt were the dolls I loved best, the dolls I conversed with in urgent whispers when I was alone.

———

Nan had been diagnosed with something called Parkinson's disease. How impressive, I thought, that Michael Parkinson, as well as being a successful television host, had discovered a disease. He must get up very early in the morning. Clearly it wasn't an infectious disease, or a grotty one that gave you spots or made bits of you fall off, like leprosy. Nan just found it hard to walk about, and she took tablets every day, and one of her hands shook a little, and that was it, really. It didn't seem to matter, not at first.

A couple of years earlier, she had moved from her house into a ground-floor flat. The flat was crammed with lovely things. There was a collection of china dogs in a battered cabinet that had once belonged to my great-granny Annie, and shaggily bellbottomed shire horses with a wooden cart that my dolls liked to ride around in. There was a ship made of shells, and a pair of tiny porcelain clogs. All were infinitely pleasing, and I played with them for hours despite having my own full-length cupboard full of toys.

I spent as much time in the flat as at home, and it was there as well as in the shop that Nan and I had our heart-to-hearts. When not talking about the distant past, we talked about the distant future; the same familiar, comforting conversations on repeat. I was going to be a writer and also an archaeologist. I'd have a house with a granny annexe so she could live with me and still have her own TV to watch

Brookside. Together we would write the story of her life into a book.

One day we were sketching out our future like this when she spoilt it.

'Ah, but when you grow up,' she said, 'you won't want to hang about with your old nan any more.'

I clutched Bethany Fleamarket to my chest a little tighter.

'You'll see,' I told Nan. 'You'll see.'

We resumed the conversation as it was supposed to go, and then she started talking about how one day I would marry a nice man, and how beautiful I would look in my big white dress with my lovely curly hair that everyone admired, and how proud she would be. She would sit in the front of the church and cry happy tears. I couldn't see why she kept bringing up my wedding, and with something like doubt in her voice. Of course she was going to be at my wedding. I was going to wear her gold necklace, threaded with tiny red roses. I hadn't planned it much beyond that. It seemed just as well not to, as I was only eight.

I cut the conversation short and went to the bathroom, where Nan had a special shower with a seat that folded out of the wall. This was another place where I could take Bethany Fleamarket and the gang and pull a curtain across to divide my world from the world outside. I began to air my grievances.

'She's talking like it's not going to happen, any of it. What does she think – I'm going to become somebody else and just swan off and leave?'

Bethany stared blankly. This was because she couldn't make facial expressions, but I could tell that she was thinking hard.

'Leave it with me,' she said eventually. 'I'll come up with something.'

Bethany's something arrived a few days later, in the form of a wizard in oversized purple robes and a floppy hat, all spattered with a haphazard arrangement of yellow stars. His wispy beard trailed all the way down to his toes. I was a little taken aback when he quite literally popped up out of nowhere in Nan's shower, but not as taken aback as I would have been if I hadn't spent the past few months in the company of Bethany Fleamarket. The wizard wouldn't tell me his name and I could never guess it. It wasn't Rumpelstiltskin: that was the first one I tried.

The anonymous wizard had been recruited to coach me in magic. Magic, in this case, meant moving dead leaves on the playground tarmac without touching them and making the green man appear as soon as I approached to cross the road – and flying, of course. Eventually I would graduate to more advanced magical abilities, and then nothing could go wrong that wouldn't be in my power to remedy with a bit of hocus-pocus.

'How's the flying coming along?' he asked me some weeks later.

'I gave it up. You know I did. It was pointless. I tried all the things you said, even running with a plastic shopping bag on a windy day, but it's just jumping. And I don't see how it helps with Nan acting strange, or school, or any-thing, really.'

'Hmmm . . .' he pondered, his brow wrinkling so hard it folded over. 'Do you still *think* about flying?'

'Sure, sometimes. I dream about it a lot. I keep having this dream that I'm soaring over the sea. It's lovely, actually. I feel free.'

His face changed so completely it was as if he'd rearranged himself. He looked a hundred years younger, and he was beaming.

'There you are, then,' he said. 'You're flying. Just because something's in your head doesn't mean it's not real.'

Morning Has Broken

What is a ghost? A tragedy condemned to repeat itself time and again? An instant of pain, perhaps. Something dead which still seems to be alive. An emotion, suspended in time. Like a blurred photograph. Like an insect trapped in amber.
Dr Casares in Guillermo del Toro's film,
The Devil's Backbone[1]

Summer 1998

The summer I was ten seemed to go on for ever. Half the novels I've read have a summer like that – long, hot, languishing, permeated by a mounting sense of dread. Maybe it's become a motif because it's recognisable. Maybe we've all had summers like that.

I had a thing about coins at the time. I dug up half my parents' garden and underneath the bushes around Nan's flat, looking for coins and whatever else might be buried in the soil. I found a large penny from 1901, worn smooth and barely legible. 1901 was the year Queen Victoria died, which meant that my coin had first belonged to a real Victorian person, probably wearing one of those really tall top hats, or a frilly mob cap. I turned the penny over and over in my fingers, as if it could summon him or her. I cleaned it with HP Sauce because I'd read you were supposed to do that, and afterwards it always smelt vaguely of bacon sandwiches.

New coins were easier to come by. My holy grail was any coin engraved with the year we were currently in. I liked to hold them, twinkling, up to the light. Happy little magpie. Then I wrapped them in tissues, wrote the date on in biro, and tucked them away in a special drawer, resting in the knowledge that they were not getting any less shiny.

I wanted to stop it, the relentless march of time, but the days kept coming and everything was changing.

—

Puberty came for me early and wasn't forgiving. There was the acne, which got steadily worse until everyone was so disgusted at the sight of me that Mum took me to the doctor, who prescribed antibiotics. Then, suddenly I grew three inches in height. I was astonished at how far away the ground was, and I kept bumping my newly widened hips into doorframes and furniture. Plum-coloured stretch marks arched across my thighs and my ever-increasing breasts.

Mum noted that the *Aladdin* crop tops I'd inherited from my cousin Danielle were no longer up to the job, and she took me to a ladies' bra shop called Contessa. Contessa was staffed by a herd of stout, pearl-clad women in later middle age, and they hollered my bra size at one another while customers politely ignored the scene unfolding in the fitting area.

one

'I CAN'T BELIEVE SHE'S ONLY TEN,' shouted the bra women, 'AND FILLING A THIRTY-SIX C.'*

'Aren't you *lucky*,' they said.

I didn't feel lucky. I felt conspicuous. It wasn't like I'd wished upon a star and had these graciously bestowed by the Boob Fairies. They just grew on the front of me at an absurdly young age.

As Mum finished paying at the till, she thanked the bra women. 'Right,' she said, turning to me. 'Come on, Busty Bertha.' I trudged three paces behind, mentally garrotting her with one of the bras.

My periods were going to start soon. Mum and Nan had each prepped me, separately, in advance. In the flat, Nan told me the story of her first period, and how she was convinced she was dying. She didn't tell anyone for months but made a will and kept it under her pillow, even though she didn't really have anything to bequeath. At home, Mum took a more practical approach and handed me some pads.

When the time came, my problem was not the anticipation of my imminent demise or a lack of menstrual products, but that there were no sanitary bins in the primary-school toilets. I sat on the loo for a full ten minutes, clutching my inexpertly wrapped, blood-soaked pad and pondering my predicament.

Eventually I tucked it up my sleeve and crept out of the cubicle. I chucked the offending item at the bin full of paper hand towels and, in my panic, I missed completely. I picked it up off the floor and tried again. That was a slam dunk, so I hurriedly splashed water on my hands and fled

---

* I'd have been better off in a 30F, but that's a discussion for another day.

the scene. Later, I had an excruciating word with my class teacher, which was overheard, of course, and the news was round the whole school by the end of the day.

Shortly afterwards, they brought sanitary bins into the girls' toilets. Just for me. My classmates referred to them as 'Laura's Bins'.

———

As I was lurching reluctantly towards womanhood, Nan was dying. The long summer stretched out in anticipation of it. *The valley of the shadow of death.*

She seemed to shrink as I grew. She gave up her knitting, then her crossword. She struggled to walk even with the Zimmer frame, shuffling with agonising slowness. It was as if she were fading away, all the colour draining out of her image. She kept having falls. She went into hospital and came out again, and then she went back in. I didn't see her for weeks, a sort of practice run. I practised not thinking about her.

I came up with whole catalogues of people that death could have instead. As if the Grim Reaper were wandering around with a scythe, taking his pick of potential victims, and I might be able to negotiate with him. He was quite welcome, for example, to Mrs Haddock, my former class teacher whose leggings, when she bent over, stretched far too thin over her ample backside. I felt that she didn't like me, and once, after I asked her to clarify a set of instructions, she replied, 'That's the problem with you, Laura: you've got no initiative.' I nursed that grudge for three years. Every time Nan and I spoke about her she had the name of a different fish: Mrs Kipper, Mrs Halibut, Mrs Rainbow Trout.

I was coming out of my after-school French class and very deliberately not thinking about Nan in hospital when I passed Mrs Haddock in the corridor. 'Aren't you a bit old for those?' she said, gesturing to the Beanie Babies I was carrying. I only had Bernie the dog, Fleece the lamb, and Chocolate the moose on me at the time, which really is hardly any Beanie Babies, and anyway, only a person who didn't understand Beanie Babies would think that it was even possible to be too old for Beanie Babies. Mrs Haddock was exactly such a person.

As soon as she was safely out of earshot, I muttered, 'Town cheese.'

That was mine and Nan's favourite insult, after a scene in *Goodbye, Mr Chips* (1939), in which faux-elderly Robert Donat (Robert Doughnut to us) breaks up a fistfight between two schoolboys. It transpires that the fight began because one boy called the other the town cheese. 'The town cheese!' exclaims Robert Doughnut from underneath his enormous eyebrows. 'That *was* ill-mannered of you, Colley.'[2]

At school, *I* was the town cheese, and if I didn't have anyone to make me feel better, I would just be the town cheese all the time, for ever, and that would be it. Who was going to come up with fish names with me if not Nan? Who was going to take my side and make me believe that I was better than them, or at least better than they thought I was? Wouldn't death consider someone, almost literally anyone, else?

I set out on a one-girl mission to find out whether there were ghosts or not. This was partly because of Nan, but not only because of her. It was a question of vital importance, one that touched almost all areas of my life. I didn't know when I had started seeing ghosts. It was like trying to recount when I first saw a pigeon. They were just *around*, and always had been. Jane Hunt still slept in my bed. But lately, I'd become suspicious that I might have been making all this up.

There was the fact that I never saw ghosts at home or in the street or in shops. Even the boney around St James' had been still and quiet for some time. I only saw ghosts at school, or when visiting Nan in hospital. This made sense: a hospital is an obvious venue for ghosts to congregate, and once someone had told me, perhaps mistakenly, that our school building had been repurposed as a military hospital during World War I. But the ghosts were never soldiers, and they never seemed sick or injured. They were children, and some of them did look suspiciously like the illustrations in my copy of *What Katy Did*.

I read everything about ghosts in the local library – reports from paranormal investigators; first-hand accounts of poltergeists and grey ladies and headless apparitions in Tudor pubs; and fiction too, everything from Goosebumps to M. R. James.* I liked that you finished a Goosebumps novel feeling extremely well informed about your ghost: you knew exactly how he died, and when, why he became a ghost, where he lived, and how he spent his free time. On the opposite end of the spectral spectrum, there was the eerie, *Oooh! There might be something over there . . . maybe . . .* , which I found equally satisfying, in a different

---

* 'The Goosebumps' books, by R. L. Stine, are a series of pre-teen horror novels with titles like *Egg Monsters From Mars* and *The Blob That Ate Everyone*. The covers featured characters' heads poking out of a lake of brightly coloured, bubbling gunge.

way. In hindsight, all this reading about ghosts may have contributed to why I saw so many of them. But I failed to establish definitively whether there were ghosts or not, and that troubled me.

'Are you real?' I asked a boy in the school cloakroom. He wore a faded sailor suit and had a long fringe of mousy hair and pale, seawater eyes. He shrugged and walked away.

'Laura, who are you talking to?' came an impatient voice behind me.

'Myself.'

———

When Nan came out of hospital, she didn't get her hair dyed. It was bright white.

'You look old,' I said, cruelly. Her white hair made me angry. I couldn't see why it should make me angry, and that made me even more angry.

'I am old,' she replied.

She was giving up. That was what made me angry. She should at least have been *trying* to get better so that we could go back to how things were. How things should be. But the falls, the hospital, the medicines, all of it had knocked the fight right out of her.

On the evening of Nan's seventy-fifth birthday, we were alone in the flat. The television was switched off, and the fringed standing lamp cast a dim glow in the corner. I perched on the arm of Nan's chair and draped myself over to lean against her. That was how we always sat, ever since having me on her lap began to hurt her knees. She was taking happy birthday phone calls. My cousins in Yorkshire sang, 'Happy birthday, dear Nanny Bett. Happy birthday to you.'

As she put the receiver back on the cradle with a loud click, she started to cry. I hovered a moment, unsure what to do, then I buried my face in her shoulder and kept very still. We stayed like that a long time.

We went to bed at nine o'clock, because we always went to bed at nine o'clock. Nan used to say that every hour of sleep before midnight is worth two after. We slept together in her double bed, and I borrowed her nighties rather than bring my own from home. That night I lay beside her, both awake and not talking. I was wearing an orange nightdress from the sixties: polyester that felt sticky in the warmth of summer, like peach juice, with a thin layer of netting over the top. I tore the netting quietly with my fingernails as the memory of her sobs reverberated around the dark room.

When the school holidays began, people descended on us. Family members from all over the world came to visit in rapid succession. The fact that these were goodbyes was unspoken. I half knew, and it nagged at me.

Nan's brother travelled all the way from New Zealand. He handed me a £20 note – equivalent to winning the ten-year-old lottery – and I looked up at him, uncomprehending. He said, 'Well, I probably won't see you again.'

One of Nan's sisters came from wherever she lived with her daughter. They sat in the front room of the flat and talked with Nan and Mum, while Danielle and I went to the bedroom to try on the matching black-and-white strappy sundresses we'd just bought from the high street. My favourite dress was becoming indecent, and I could see that Mum was itching to whisk it out of the wardrobe. Here was a potential replacement. I stared at myself in the mirror on Nan's wardrobe door, taken aback by the curve of my hips, the fabric stretched tight over my chest. I looked older than Danielle.

I saw Mum thinking along similar lines as we returned in our new dresses. I felt I should sit on the sofa, instead of draped across Nan as usual, but all seats were occupied. I stood about awkwardly.

On my way back from the toilet, I stopped, just out of sight, to listen to Nan boast of my latest school report. She moved on seamlessly to my poem about a tree that had been published in the local newspaper two years before. She kept copies in her magazine rack to show to people. I was relishing the words 'ever so clever' and the pride in her voice when my great-aunt interjected, 'She's too clever for her own good, Bett. She's a funny thing. No one's going to want her if she carries on as she is.'

I heard notes of indignation as I took myself back to the bathroom. I sat on the toilet lid and stared hard at the shower seat. I wanted Bethany Fleamarket but she was at home. Our wizard had been making himself scarce for a while.

'Come *on*,' I urged the empty air.

And *pop*.

He was a little hazy that day, and greyer. A sketch of himself, more cartoonish than usual. But he was all there, and visibly agitated, hopping nimbly from one foot to the other.

'About time.'

'Don't complain, Laura. It doesn't suit you.'

I scowled at him.

He said, 'If you want things to be different, make them different.'

'But sometimes you can't make it different. It just is. What then?'

He stroked his beard, eyes shining like two silver coins beneath his raggedy grey eyebrows.

'Ah yes, what then?'

'Put up with it?' I suggested.

'Wrong. Wrong, wrong, wrong,' he sang, chiming like a bell. He spun round in a circle and pointed a finger at me. 'You're wrong.'

I threw up my hands in a gesture of hopelessness, and he mimicked my gesture. He had been particularly annoying of late.

'You imagine it different?'

'Right. If you imagine it, then it is.'

'Is it, though?'

'I'm here, aren't I?'

'I think so?'

'Precisely. Look, do you want to save her or don't you?'

'I don't know if I *can* save her.'

I didn't see him vanish. He was just gone.

———

By the autumn Nan was back in hospital. I sensed that she was having a bad time, and that my parents were shielding me from the worst. I didn't see her at all in those final weeks. I got up each morning and went to school, and I felt the threads between us, tugging.

On the first Sunday in October, I climbed the war memorial in the park and looked out, red-gold leaves all round me and conkers littered over the ground. My little brother was gathering them into a bag while Dad talked on his mobile phone. His voice was low and unusually serious. I strained to hear. As he pressed the button to end the call, he spoke louder – to me. I thought he was going to tell me to get down from there, but instead he said, 'It won't be long now.'

I felt brushed by something black and unknowable to come. Something was circling, swooping lower and lower. It was a sense that there were things in my future that I didn't yet know existed, and they were not nice things.

Nan was going to die soon, I understood that much. I could feel Dad bracing himself against the impact. All the grown-ups were doing it, a collective flinching. It was in the strained, tight-lipped faces and the muttered conversations. It was in the late-night trips to hospital. This was going to happen, and it was going to hurt.

The days after she died were a blur. For the first time in my life, I found myself longing to go to school, but I couldn't go to school because it was half-term. My uncle came down from Yorkshire for the funeral with his wife and eight children in tow. In the scramble to house everyone, Mum and her siblings pooled the children and stepchildren they had between them (sixteen total, twelve present at the time) and grouped us by age and gender. This meant that Danielle and Jessica (both twelve), Kirsty (fourteen), and I went to stay with Auntie Pat and Uncle Bobby.

We lucked out. Auntie Pat and Uncle Bobby had no children of their own and they took great pleasure in spoiling their nieces. Every evening we picked a film from Blockbuster, along with popcorn and pipes of Pringles galore. It was a glorious extended girlie sleepover and I felt grown up to be included. Kirsty and Jessica taught us a new card game called Cheat, and that was a riot. I found I could just put my grief aside. There was no room for it, crammed in as we were. It was only at night, lying on cushions on the floor by the radiator, that I stared into the dark and thought of Nan, but I didn't cry.

Nothing was ever the same again. The flat was sold. The shop was sold, then demolished, and most of St Mary Street with it. My relationship with the rest of the family began to feel increasingly strained. It was as if Nan had been the sun, and we'd all been in orbit. After she died, we each spun off separately into our own grief.

A few months ago, I was going through boxes in the attic, and I found the gifts I'd bought with my pocket money to go around Nan's hospital bed. There was a pill-box on which was painted a boxer dog that looked just like one in Great-Granny Annie's cabinet, and an orange-and-yellow plush sunflower with a looped string so that it could be hung from the bedframe. And there were dozens of coins wrapped in tissues with the date written on. All these things I had kept in an effort to preserve what was already lost. The black-and-white strappy dress was there too. It was the dress I wore to Nan's funeral.

Holding the slippery synthetic fabric between my fingers brought it all back: the wet stench of the flowers, the stone floor of the chapel, the opening bars of 'Morning Has Broken', tears dripping off the end of my dad's nose. Everything had broken. The vicar droned on and on, sounding half asleep, and he talked of heaven as if Nan were floating on a cloud playing a harp. He had so clearly never met her. She'd be asking St Peter for a vodka and Coke. 'There's a love. You're so good at making them.'

I knew I was supposed to be saying goodbye, selecting my solemn final words, but all I could whisper was, '*Please find a way to come back to me.*'

Body Language

Give me a girl at an impressionable age, and she is mine for life.

Muriel Spark, *The Prime of Miss Jean Brodie*[1]

Spring 2001

I decided I would go somewhere nobody knew me. I would reinvent myself. A fresh start.

The move to secondary school offered a golden opportunity. I would find a school that was completely different from my current school, and more like the schools in the Enid Blyton and Chalet School books I loved so much.* I was happier when immersed in a book than at any other time. Surely, if I went to a school that was like schools in books, I would meet people who were more like me. I could create a new life for myself, a life where I fitted in. So I got hold of prospectuses, filled in application forms, went to interviews, and swotted and blagged my way into

---

* The Chalet School is a series of school story novels by Elinor M. Brent-Dyer, originally published between 1925 and 1970.

a free place at a private girls' school out in the Hampshire countryside.

I loved it there: the tuck shop, morning prayers, my initials embroidered on my bottle-green netball skirt – all that lovely, leafy privilege. It was my Malory Towers. In my mind, there was little difference between a fictional 1940s boarding school and a modern, fee-paying day school for middle-class daughters. After all, they were both posh. It became a running joke at home to pronounce the name of my new school in the most drawling, affected accent possible. Mum and I could run the first syllable to four or five seconds.

The school buses were supplied by a coach company and so we were driven around in coaches that had *PRINCESS* emblazoned across the side. I seemed to be the only one who thought this was funny. In my first term, Libby Matthews remarked that I 'talked like *EastEnders*' and I was gently nudged into extracurricular speech and drama classes. The tutor praised my ability to project my voice to the back of the hall and I knew enough not to mention market stalls, but still she added, 'Try to pronounce *all* the letters in each word, sweetie.' I started to overcompensate by talking like the queen, but I could only keep that up part-time and the results, in retrospect, must have been hilarious.

Mostly I adored my teachers. I'll never forget Dr Sheppard, who taught us physics and was the first person I'd known who had a Ph.D. Initially I'd thought he was a GP who'd got lost or something. When I learned that Dr Sheppard shared my interest in archaeology, I started talking to him about it in my usual, rather intense way, and one day he brought me a carrier bag full of actual

Roman coins as a gift. I kept thinking it must have been a mistake. Surely he wasn't *giving* me these? To *keep*? I trawled the local library and our Microsoft Encarta CD-ROM to identify and date them all, sketched and catalogued them, wrapped each one in its handwritten description. 'Are you *sure* you don't want them back?' I asked. He didn't want them back.

What I loved most of all was my new surroundings. There were two main buildings: one was brand-new and purpose-built, housing the school hall and most of our classrooms, with blossoming trees outside the windows and bunny rabbits on the lawns. The other was a red-brick Elizabethan manor house. I ached with delight at its oak-panelled rooms, coats of arms, carved roses and fleurs-de-lys, its window seats and huge open fireplaces. It even had turrets like a castle. We had our music lessons there, and our drama lessons in the long gallery upstairs. The head-mistress's offices occupied much of the ground floor, along with reception, another music room, and the 'san' (short for sanatorium), where Matron kept a bed made up for any girls who were indisposed.

The manor house came with a Tudor sunken garden, where a rare species of orchid grew. Occasionally orchid enthusiasts would visit, with big cameras and little note-books, crouching respectfully beside the flowers. Between the two school buildings were lawns where we would laze about in twos and threes with revision for summer exams, and a fountain, which sixth-formers filled with soap bub-bles and rubber ducks on the last day of summer term. An avenue of lime trees lined the front drive on either side, and sometimes sheep would graze there. I'd stop to chat to them halfway round the country run. We even had a school dog, a cocker spaniel-cross-Dalmatian, whom we collectively worshipped and competed to take for walks.

The best places on the school site were those that were out of bounds. The whole third floor of the manor house was off-limits before it was converted into the new sixth form, and I used to tiptoe up the winding staircase, holding my breath as I stepped on each floorboard in case it should collapse beneath me. I spent many happy hours creeping among the dustsheets. There were bars on the upper windows, which prompted me to read up on the history of the building. In the nineteenth century our manor house had been a lunatic asylum. What had people seen, I wondered; what had people felt in those same rooms?

The sunken garden, with its ancient, crumbling steps, was too visible to trespass on very often, but occasionally I would chance it. I loved to think that I was placing my feet exactly where some long-forgotten Elizabethan lady had put hers. I saw her in a ruff and heavy brocade gown, pearl earrings, and dainty slippers. A little dog ran at her heels. Once I took off my shoes and socks, so that my footsteps could commune more fully with hers.

Behind the playing fields was woodland where bluebells erupted every spring. It was easiest of all to sneak off there. If the other girls questioned it, I told them casually that I had taken up smoking. I liked to wander among the trees and the ivy, dreaming, spotting glimpses of deer, heading as far back as I could to where the trees thinned out and where starkly, in the clearing, there stood an enormous electricity pylon. It felt like the end of the world.

—

How could I be unhappy at this magnificent school? There was nothing obviously wrong. In many ways, I was having the time of my life. I was form prefect. I won inter-school competitions for Latin, for public speaking, and for maths. I passed violin exams and drama exams. I was tripping over prizes and certificates. And yet it was clear, once I'd been at the school a while, that I'd dragged my problem – whatever it was – along with me. I was no longer bullied, but I was still out of step with everyone, as clumsy interpersonally as I was physically.

I started revising for the summer exams at Christmas, going over everything we'd done in the first term while memorising everything from the next two terms as we covered it: an hour every evening, increasing to three, in a neatly written-up timetable. There was no need for this. Standards were higher than at my old school, but the work came naturally to me, and I would have done well regardless. I just had to do something to stave off the fear.

I got to know Matron quite well, spending more and more time in the san with asthma attacks and mystery headaches, and I was struggling to sleep. I'd stare at the ceiling, stare at the clock, stare at the ceiling, stare at the clock, back and forth as hours passed. I watched the smoky hours swirl between fitful, fragmented dreams. The dreams twisted and turned and always took me back to Nan's flat. I stood outside the locked door and peered in at the kitchen window. Her face would appear and then vanish. Sometimes I found the door open, went inside, and carefully locked us both in. Sometimes she wasn't herself.

'Are you real?' I asked her. 'Are you a ghost? Will you stay?'

Mum took me to the doctor, who prescribed zopiclone,

sleeping pills like tiny blue moons. He warned that they were addictive. I was only supposed to take them every other day, but, lying sleep-starved and desperate in the small hours, I would inevitably cave and pop an extra one. Soon I couldn't sleep at all without them. Then I had to take two. Then I ran out and had to wait. In the morning I slathered Maybelline Dream Matte Mousse into the dark, hollowed-out space beneath my eyes.

I wasn't miserable every moment. The misery came in sharp stabs that took my breath away. I became so terribly frightened and angry and despairing, sometimes for a superficial reason which seemed enormous and sometimes for no reason at all. I just *hurt*. I'd thought that moving schools would fix things – and it did, until it didn't. So, I burrowed inward, berating myself, scrawling pages and pages in various diaries and notebooks. I couldn't confide in anyone else because it was all wrapped up in a secret.

I had taken to scratching my forearms with whatever I could find – sharpened pencils, drawing pins, scissors, the corner of anything metal or plastic – and this became the answer to everything. It calmed me. It subdued the unnameable, unbearable tumult enough that I could keep studying and smiling and doing whatever was required. The pain focused my mind, humming and vibrating with its own pain, somewhere near the ceiling. It brought me back to my body. At the same time, damaging my body released me from the sense that I was trapped within it. My skin, the barrier between me and the rest of the world, could be broken.

It was also a way to punish myself for any failure, and to enact and exorcise the fury that overtook me from nowhere. If I was overwhelmed, it would fix that too. The bleeding and bruising on my arms constituted far more eloquent self-expression than the mountains of shit poetry I was writing. It depicted how damaged I felt, and I fantasised about letting people see while hiding it meticulously. Hurting myself scratched every itch, ticked every box, solved every problem. I was bulletproof: there was nothing I couldn't withstand, no hurt I could not erase in an instant with a hurried flick of my wrist, like lighting a match. I came to think of my habit as almost a separate entity, as a friend and a refuge.

At first, I barely bled. Just scratches, little white lines. But the secrecy, the deceit, the sneaking about fed and fattened the beast and soon it filled my life. I was averaging five sessions a day, the scratches had deepened to cuts, and I thought about hurting myself every single minute. I filled both arms and both thighs and had to get creative: the soles of my feet, the back of my neck, careful placement on my hands that could be passed off as an accident. I was sick with the fear of being discovered. I dreamed of it every night and woke up sweating and shaking – and I knew it was inevitable.

I believed I had invented self-harm. I thought my mind was the first in human history to propose this bizarre solution to unhappiness. How sick, how intricately deranged must I be.

The clock, I knew, was ticking.

———

The day I was found out was a Monday. I was running late for PE. I was appalling at sports, and I had the stereotypical PE teacher – tanned, athletic, shouty. I used to change into my kit in the toilets, pleading self-consciousness, so that when the feared one erupted into the locker room and hollered us out in our hockey socks, I'd have just made it back in time to slam my locker shut and fumble for the key.

That day, there wasn't time to go anywhere. All the others were at least half changed, some already tying laces on their trainers. For a second, I weighed up the risk of being shouted at against the risk of the cuts on my arms and legs being noticed by the other girls. The latter outcome was far worse, but the former was a certainty if I scuttled off to the loo. I'd probably be left behind altogether. Everyone seemed engrossed in getting dressed, so I unbuttoned my shirt and, as quickly as I could manage, swapped the shirt for a t-shirt and grabbed my tracksuit top.

'WHAT HAPPENED TO YOUR ARMS?' yelled Libby Matthews beside me.

In slow motion, every girl in that locker room turned and stared.

I gabbled something without knowing what I said.

The zip on my tracksuit was deafening.

And then somehow the moment had passed. We were all in our PE kits, the teacher was there, and we filed out. Walking over to the sports hall was like wading through water, my footsteps on gravel oddly amplified.

There was a lot of whispering behind hands over breaktime. Libby followed me around the school, demanding answers.

'What happened to you, seriously? Did you do that to *yourself*? You *did* do that to yourself, didn't you? Why would you even do that? *Why do you cut yourself, Laura?*'

She kept shoving her stupid freckly face in front of my

face, but I dodged and answered every question with, 'Fuck off, Libby.'

Eventually she got bored and went back to draping herself over desks and chairs, chatting with her pals as she ironed her waist-length hair with straightening rods that fizzled and steamed.

Hours passed. The tight knot of terror in my chest began to loosen just a little. I reasoned that the other girls were nosy, but they were also self-absorbed. They would gossip and then they would move on to the next thing. This might be okay.

It wasn't okay.

Georgie sat next to me in geography and passed a note, expressing concern. I was penning a reply on my lap beneath the desk when Mrs Cole appeared in the doorway. Mrs Cole was a senior tutor, ranking below the deputy head but above the department heads in that peculiar school hierarchy. She was past retirement age, thin, and frail-looking, and only came into school part-time.

'Could I borrow Laura Richmond, please?'

There was a long pause. I scrunched the note into my fist and stood up. It was clear what this was about – to me and to everyone in the room. I considered making a run for it, but Mrs Cole was blocking the doorway and, anyway, the game was up. I followed her through the corridor. My feet were heavy, palms tingling.

She led me silently to her office, closed the door, and gestured for me to sit opposite her. I perched on the edge of the chair, as if ready to dash from the room.

I folded my arms across my chest and denied everything – until she told me to roll up my sleeves. Then I admitted it but refused to say more, firing monosyllables in response to every question she asked. I was cornered. I would at least go down fighting.

Looking back, I don't think Mrs Cole wanted to fight me. She might have wanted to help. Perhaps she was trying to be kind, even to encourage me to confide in her. There would have been no telling that to this thirteen-year-old, with cuts and bruises all over her and nothing but panic behind her eyes. I was cold and sarcastic and rude to Mrs Cole, as I would be rude to many other well-meaning people over the next few years.

As she admitted defeat, she said sadly, 'I've never seen anyone so defensive and so aggressive at the same time.' She handed me over to the deputy head.

Miss Miller, brisk in twinset and pearls, reached across her desk for the telephone. 'I'll speak to your mother.'

I heard my own voice, cool and measured. 'I'd prefer to speak to her myself if you don't mind.'

There was a pause.

I added, 'She should hear it from me.'

Miss Miller hesitated, her hand still hovering over the phone.

'You will tell her tonight. And I'll call your parents first thing tomorrow morning.'

There followed a series of agonising conversations – with my mum, with the nurse at the doctor's surgery, with the doctor himself, with the counsellor I was sent to see, and then his replacement, and then her replacement, then various social workers, and their replacements, ad nauseam. I was presented to person after person in this way, to discuss things I couldn't articulate. No one seemed to know what to do with me. The doctor prescribed antidepressants. The counsellors wanted me to hold ice cubes instead of self-harming. They wanted me to flick an elastic band on my wrist. They wanted me to draw on myself in red pen. They were missing the point by so far – by light years, the entire expanse of the universe sitting vast and vacant between me and them – that I simply didn't know what to say in response. I dealt with this barrage of new people and toe-curling interviews by hurting myself more enthusiastically than ever.

At school, the whispering behind hands let up, although not because the girls had lost interest so much as because some of them had started cutting themselves too. They confided in me about it. 'You're right, you know, it really helps,' said Georgie, telling me how she'd 'cut' for the first time after a row with her mum. I was sympathetic, but uncomfortable with the idea that I had somehow unwittingly recommended this course of action. I'd hurt myself for months, alone and in secret. I certainly never intended that anyone else should join in. The irony was not lost on me that after so many years as a near-pariah, suddenly I was a trendsetter – and for this.

Twelve days after my secret was out, I was summoned to see Miss Miller – not in her office at the main school building, but at the manor house. It was a bleak, drizzly morning. I presented myself at reception in my damp blazer and was directed, instead, straight to the headmistress.

Mrs Wentworth's office was not so much an office as a suite of rooms, furnished with armchairs and low, studded Chesterfield sofas in oxblood leather, lines of bookshelves, and a long table for meetings. If you were called in under favourable circumstances, there were plates of biscuits laid out. As I knocked and peered around the half-open door, I noted there was not a biscuit in sight.

Mrs Wentworth had once been a PE teacher. She was old school. Jolly hockey sticks. Play the game, pull those socks up, et cetera. She had covered our netball lesson the previous term and I still hadn't forgiven her for crowing, 'Goal defence is *lazy*,' as I half-heartedly attempted to intercept the ball. I was caught between disliking her and craving her approval – and here we were, face to face, alone for the first time in that boudoir of an office.

'I don't know how you can do it,' she said, making a face like she was chewing on a wasp. 'How you can ... *cut yourself* like that.'

She mimed it, cringing. 'I would be too squeamish.'

She may not have known how I could do it, but she certainly seemed to know why. She presented me with a catalogue of reasons.

Firstly, I was 'obviously' doing it for attention. It didn't seem to matter that I'd carefully hidden it from everyone for so many months, that it had been brought to public notice without my consent, and that I'd give anything for it to be a secret again. It was ironic that what was essentially a means of dealing with my emotions 'in-house' so that I didn't have to bother anyone else with them – admittedly more motivated by cowardice than altruism – was read as an invitation for everyone to wade in. So much for attention-seeking. If she'd accused me of attention-dodging, she might have had a point. Besides, even if I *were* doing it for attention, if I were prepared to go to those lengths—

The rising vehemence in her voice cut off my train of thought. She was still listing reasons.

I was doing it to get out of lessons.

I was doing it because normal life wasn't exciting enough, so I had to 'glam it up' a bit.

I was doing it because I was a drama queen.

As she went on and on, I pictured an asteroid – or perhaps the back end of a space rocket – in flames, hurtling down through the sky.

Smoke trailing upwards from a pleasingly headmistress-shaped crater.

It would be a shame about the manor house but, on balance, worth it.

'Don't you realise how lucky you are?' she continued. 'There are girls all over the world who would kill to have your life, your education, your opportunities ...'

I winced at the reminder of my 'charity girl' status at this fee-paying school.

She built to a crescendo. 'There are children starving in Africa!'

How was that relevant? Was I supposed to be cutting myself out of insufficient gratitude that I wasn't starving in Africa? Nan used to say that there were children starving in Africa when I didn't want to finish my dinner. I wasn't going to post my leftover sausage and beans to Africa, so what did it matter whether I ate them or not? It hadn't occurred to me that Nan couldn't bear to waste food because she had once been hungry, but it dawned on me then, for the first time, in front of Mrs Wentworth. The correlation between children starving in Africa and how I had found that sharp scratches were a useful means of calming myself down was still not apparent to me, but in that moment, I was convinced. I didn't need to understand to know that I was wrong.

As Mrs Wentworth carried on, I stewed and simmered in my own shame. It was sickening that I just couldn't hack it. I, with my nice school and nice family and nice life, not remotely starving in Africa . . . What was my fucking problem?

She concluded the lecture with an ultimatum. If I didn't stop this ridiculous behaviour immediately, I would be expelled.

I couldn't stop it if I wanted to. I knew that much. I resolved to hide it better.

The cold rain was a relief as I stepped outside and made my way back to lessons. Entering the classroom, I smiled brightly at the biology teacher.

'Ah, Laura, you're here . . .'

Maplewood

*If the copious writings of the mad are about one thing, it is
above all the desire to cease to be misunderstood.*

Roy Porter, *The Faber Book of Madness*[1]

Winter 2002–3

I wasn't expelled. Instead I was sent to a psychiatrist.

If you've ever been to a psychiatrist, usually you'll
have received a letter in the post after every appointment.
This letter is not addressed to you: it's from the psychiatrist
to the GP – about you. You are copied in. Clinic letters are
a literary genre of their own, with a specific format and
vocabulary. They're full of observations and judgements
about you: your appearance, your behaviour, how mad or
sane you're considered to be at that moment in time.*

These letters always seemed to come when I was having
a good day. I'd pop downstairs, or come in from being
out – and there, on the doormat, in a specific shape and

---

* See the fabulous *Dear GP* zine of patient-authored clinic letters – 'subjective
one-sided analysis is for everyone!' deargp.home.blog

shade of envelope, the letter would be waiting. Its contents were not usually malicious; they were just not accurate, a mistranslation of what I'd said. I felt ever more disconnected from my outward persona, from my body and the sphere in which it moved. If I were invisible and everyone saw this other Laura in my place, did I even exist?

Letter in hand, the image that came to me was of an underground vault, like in films where the protagonist has dodged all the lasers and got past the thick metal walls that slide apart at the touch of a button. Inside there's a little room where whatever valuable object they're seeking is kept under a glass case. They retrieve it and flee as alarms go off and doors slide out of walls, slamming shut one by one – *thud, thud, thud.* I couldn't shake the feeling that someone was trapped in that room, but when I tried to picture them there, all I could sense was a distant trace of panic and a stuttering image of fingernails against steel, a trickle of blood.

I would throw the letter away and try to forget about it, but the phrases would circle in my head, and everything would taste odd for a few days.

I wrote a clinic letter of my own.

Dear Doctor,

I reviewed Dr Haslam on 07/11/2002. He joined my caseload after the departure of zealous Christian Steve – 'I'm a registered mental nurse and it sounds like I'm a nurse and I'm mental, har har' – and the arrival of his replacement, Sue. Dr Haslam did not seem to fully understand why he was there. He claimed that Sue had 'invited' him – as if this were her disappointing sixtieth birthday party. He did not bring alcohol to the appointment.

There are ongoing concerns about Dr Haslam's ability to care for himself and to observe basic hygiene. His body odour is a heady combination of perspiration and milk left out of the fridge. Furthermore, during this appointment, he broke wind audibly no fewer than four times, while he avoided my gaze by staring intently at the notes he was making. This — coupled with his physique, which resembles a hairy binbag filled with blancmange, spilling out between the buttons of his shirt — leads me to conclude that his diet is poor. He would benefit from occupational therapy input and perhaps a garden hose.

During assessment, Dr Haslam demonstrated confused thinking, lack of insight, and a tenuous grip on reality. Although I am quite clearly a fourteen-year-old girl, he has prescribed enough antipsychotic medication to tranquillise a woolly mammoth. When I expressed reluctance to continue the risperidone and quetiapine due to their complete ineffectiveness and disabling side effects, he advised that the doses should be increased. Over the course of two appointments, he has claimed that I suffer from bipolar disorder, psychotic depression, and schizo-affective disorder. When I suggested it seems unlikely that I would have all of these at once, he waved his hands vaguely and broke wind again. I gave brief replies to his enquiries as I was trying to hold my breath.

As we concluded the appointment, he informed me that I am to be admitted to a psychiatric hospital, saying, 'I think you'll like it there.'

In light of the upcoming admission, it is not known whether I will have further opportunity to monitor Dr Haslam.

I remain concerned about his mental state and the likelihood that he will inflict harm upon others.

Yours sincerely,
Laura Richmond

That was my first psychiatrist.

I'd had such high hopes. As I was shunted between the GP, counsellors, mental health nurses, social workers, and whoever else, it was obvious that no one really knew what my problem was or how to help. What I needed was to get past all those people and reach someone with the right expertise. A psychiatrist would be just such a person. A psychiatrist would look at me and know what he was seeing. He'd produce a bunch of keys, select the right one, wind me up, and set me going on the track to sanity. Then I would be like everyone else, and I wouldn't feel like shit any more. When Sue arranged for me to see Dr Haslam at the tall concrete building in the city centre that I'd been attending uselessly for months and months, I was relieved. Finally, I was getting somewhere.

I told him everything – all about the sleeplessness, the self-harm and decidedly amateur suicide attempts, the critical inner voices, how I wasn't always sure what was real and what I'd imagined. He swiftly prescribed anti-psychotic medications to add to my latest antidepressant and booked a further appointment to review my response.

A month or two later, we sat down again in the same room, and I told him that I couldn't take these tablets any more. I described how I'd fallen asleep at the bank, and how the woman working there thought I was drunk on a Saturday morning, frog-marched me out into the street, and left me on a bench. I told him about the nosebleeds that wouldn't stop. I told him that I'd gone into a toilet cubicle at school and lifted my jumper to find my blouse and bra soaked, and that I'd realised with horror that I was *lactating*.

'These medicines often need a period of adjustment. It should settle down. Actually, it might help to increase the dose. That way, you'll get used to it quicker. Any improvement in your symptoms?'

'Not . . . really.'

'Are you still hearing the voices?'

'Well, I don't hear them, exactly. They're thoughts. They just don't seem to come from me.'

That was when he told me that I would be going to Maplewood House. 'I think you'll like it there.'

———

Reader, I did not like it there.

The day I went in, it was snowing. Outside the front entrance was a series of huge stone spheres piled on top of one another, like marbles in front of Polly Pocket's Mental Hospital. As the snow settled, they began to resemble a stack of iced Christmas puddings. I watched them until someone came to let us in, and Mum ushered me through the doors and out of the cold. We were shown around, but I couldn't take my eyes off the windows: flurries of great whirling white flakes, the ground disappearing, the world outside muffled and muted as if the sky had fallen in. I was handed a biro and told to sign my consent to treatment. I watched my own loopy, schoolgirl signature appear on the page.

Maplewood was newly built, its facilities considered

state-of-the-art. If you were given a tour, as I was with my parents when we arrived, you would marvel at how civilised, how enlightened it all was. The beige carpets and checked curtains were almost homely. Each patient had his or her own bedroom. There was a school building, a sports hall, and a gym. We had a girls' lounge and a boys' lounge, with sofas, coffee tables, a television, and a cabinet full of books and board games. There was a separate, soundproof area to function as a sort of intensive care for anyone considered too mental even for the mental hospital. Next to that was something called a *Snoezelen*, where there were twinkly lights and lava lamps, and you were allowed to put on an Enya CD.

Surely this was where the real help was kept. The people who worked here would have the expertise to understand what was wrong with me and how to fix it. They would teach me what to do so that I didn't feel this way. Perhaps there would be better meds. I was so keen to co-operate with this process that, on being introduced to my 'named nurse' – what they called the member of staff expected to take a special interest, like a godparent but for being mental – I presented the poor man with a full catalogue of my creative writing so that he would be better equipped to analyse me. 'I'm better at writing than talking, you see,' I added apologetically as I looked at his face and saw that he was baffled. I hoped to be guided to some sort of breakthrough, so that, when I left, everything would make more sense and I wouldn't hurt like this any more. I would be on the famous road to recovery, yellow bricks stretching over the hill and far away.

Maplewood catered primarily for girls with anorexia who had reached dangerously low weights. Around two-thirds of us were in this category. They were known as pegs for 'positive eating group'. Patients were YPs, for 'young people' (although I found later that the staff didn't take kindly to being referred to as OPs). Our lives revolved around the refeeding programme, with the half-dozen of us who were not anorexic just sort of hanging around while they went through an endless cycle of weigh-ins, meals, post-meal supervision, snacks, post-snack supervision, and weigh-ins again. Clearly it was torture, and yet I was a little frightened of the pegs. They were so white and gaunt and unreal-looking. At night I heard them creeping out of bed to do star jumps.

We ate our meals in a large room with a school-dinners-style serving hatch at one end, and a long rectangular table for the pegs at the other. Smaller tables for the non-pegs were arranged in between. All the pegs had to sit around the big table until every one of them had consumed every crumb of everything they were given to eat. It wasn't unusual for the rest of us to arrive for lunch and find them still there from breakfast. If they were on 'doubles', that could be 4,500 calories every twenty-four hours. I was careful to sit with my back to the pegs because they would have to finish everything even if it was making them reflexively vomit onto the plate. We kept the radio on loud, Daniel Bedingfield's 'Gotta Get Thru This' drowning out the sound of gagging four feet behind me.

The doctors and nurses controlled every aspect of our lives. This included if and when we could see our parents, if we went to the school on-site and what we did there, how and when we could socialise with other YPs, what we ate, if and how we could exercise, and our medication. There were stark differences in treatment for favoured and non-favoured patients. Some of us were allowed phone calls, parents visiting, even to go home on weekend leave. It wasn't clear how these privileges were earned. Sometimes they were granted, sometimes not. I learned to accept it as arbitrary, like the weather.

There were so many rules, endless rules, more rules than I could ever discover by breaking them, and certainly more than I could ever remember. Often there was no discernible logic behind them. Some rules were universal; others were different for each of us. Some rules were permanent; others would fluctuate based on what had been decided, and you might or might not be informed of the changes. Usually, I didn't know a rule had changed until I was already in trouble for breaking it. There seemed to be no way of telling in advance whether whatever I was about to do or say would be deemed 'inappropriate', whether I would cross that invisible line and what the consequences would be.

One lunchtime I went up to the chilled cabinet by the serving hatch to get a yoghurt. I didn't particularly want a yoghurt, but one of the pegs was sobbing directly behind me, and I'd learned by then that there was nothing I could do for her. I would at least get away from the sound for thirty seconds. I was rewarded with the pleasing novelty of a different yoghurt from the ones we usually had. The world shrinks when you're locked up, and such things take on new significance. Even better, it was one of those that are divided into two triangles, where one has the yoghurt in and the other contains sweet crunchy stuff, so that you can tip crunchy stuff into your yoghurt as the mood takes you. Lovely. It's a yoghurt and, if you think about it, it's also occupational therapy.

A thin-lipped nurse approached in swift, purposeful

strides and informed me that I should not be eating that yoghurt. Those yoghurts were for the pegs. She glared at me as if I had known full well, as if I'd set out to sabotage the eating disorder treatment just for the hell of it. I removed the spoon from my mouth and protested that there was no indication on these yoghurts that they were *for* anyone. Someone should have put a label on them or something. It wasn't fair to have a go at me because no one had thought to do so, and there wasn't anything I could do since I'd already eaten half. The resulting scene was so overblown, so ridiculous – and it was that nurse every bit as much as me. You weren't supposed to argue back. They came down hard on you when you did.

The injustice – that I was perpetually in disgrace when I'd never intended to do anything wrong, and no one believed me when I told them so – drove me wild on a daily basis. At school I was a model pupil. In my parents' desk drawer at home were ten years of reports describing me as 'a pleasure to teach'. My brother used to parody them: 'I would like to meet Laura socially for a drink,' and so on. That's not to say that I never misbehaved, but if I did, I did so on purpose and had the sense to conceal it. Why was it so easy to be good at school and yet impossible to be good in hospital?

Another time I lost my rag was in the meds queue, standing behind Millie as she was handed her tablets through the hatch between the downstairs corridor and the clinic room where all the drugs were kept. Millie was one of the pegs. She was only twelve. As she passed back the tiny cardboard cup, the nurse said, 'Good girl. You're putting on weight so nicely. Look, you're really *rounding out.'* Millie turned away and her eyes, sunken and brimming with tears, met mine.

I had a bit of a shout about the cruelty of it and, when the resulting ruckus had died down, I found Millie, curled up underneath her bed and crying quietly. I wanted to elbow my way under there and join in. Instead, I said, 'Hey. Listen. She's talking shite. She's just being horrible because she can.' Millie didn't reply.

Every evening we had the 6.15 Meeting. Privately I called it the 6.15 Bollocking. All staff on shift and all YPs were required to congregate in the girls' lounge. No one was keen, partly because 6.15 was halfway through *The Simpsons* and partly because of all the bollocking. The most common offence for us to 'discuss' was 'inappropriate language'. 'What does that *even mean?*' I wailed. I knew what it meant. It meant swearing is not allowed. Bullshit. There are situations – such as finding yourself incarcerated in an actual mental hospital – when swearing is absolutely an appropriate response. Arguably, it would be inappropriate *not* to swear under such circumstances.

I've loved to swear ever since I was little, and Nan had no qualms about swearing in my presence. 'Bugger this for a game of soldiers,' she would say, pulling the lever on her chair and lowering herself gingerly onto stiff legs. When something surprised her, she adopted an awed tone and half whispered, 'Well, bugger me …' She used to impersonate my long-deceased great-granny Annie with an exasperated, 'What with the kids and the cats and the *bloody* lodgers!' There was a fantastic crescendo on the *bloody*, which you can apply to any rant, and it rounds it off beautifully – if, like me, you are inappropriate.

I maintain that swearing is one of the most harmless

of life's pleasures. It's free. It's legal. It doesn't rot your teeth. It doesn't give you cancer. It doesn't raise your cholesterol or your blood pressure. It might even lower your blood pressure. If you're severely distressed, as we all were at Maplewood, and pronouncing a torrent of expletives gives you the tiniest relief, then I say fucking go for it. Call it self-care – not that self-care had been invented then.

Vocalising this argument also turned out to be inappropriate. I wondered if there had been an appropriateness meeting, to which I had not been invited. I imagined everyone else in the world – or all the staff in that hospital – seated around a table. The consultant psychiatrist would have the *Oxford English Dictionary* in his hands and would open the first page. 'Right, aardvarks. What do we think? Are aardvarks appropriate? We can't have them roaming the hospital, but will we permit the YPs to mention them?' Everyone would have two cards, labelled 'appropriate' and 'inappropriate', and would hold them up to vote.

Admittedly the 6.15 public bollockings became more and more deserved. Since I couldn't be good, no matter how hard I tried, I found that it hurt less if I gave up trying. With no conscious planning, I started to break rules on purpose, to become the miscreant and troublemaker that they all believed me to be. I might as well enjoy myself in advance of the inevitable bollocking. But I was lying if I said I didn't care. I cut myself with razor blades hidden inside my mattress after every showdown with the nurses, concealing bloody tissues inside screwed-up paper before binning them. I did it to congratulate myself when I got away with something as well as to console myself when I didn't. Everything became a means of clinging to autonomy when I was stuck indefinitely on a locked ward.

I realised for the first time that long walks are essential to the maintenance of my brain. I walk fast, alone, with music, daydreaming vividly, and this seems to function as an aid to processing new information in much the way that sleep does. Restricted to a confined space, I became more agitated and less able to manage interacting with other people. I paced up and down the upstairs corridor, along the rows of bedroom doors, bouncing from stairwell to stairwell and memorising every inch of wall and door and floor and radiator and skirting board. I imagined myself twirling in a field like Maria von Trapp, like a snowflake on the wind, miles and miles of open space all around me. When I was caught sprinting along the upstairs corridor, just to raise my heart rate, to make myself breathless – an illusion of fresh air – I had to sit in the girls' lounge with the pegs on post-meal supervision. I had to sit and be watched.

I liked to imagine breaking out, scaling the high wire fence like a cat, leaping deftly over the coils of barbed wire at the top and sustaining barely a scratch. 'Give me liberty,' I would cry, 'or give me death!' I'd sprint the wrong way down the motorway, dodging cars as I went. The police would catch up with me eventually, but they'd be so impressed by my pluck that they would drive me to the train station and distract the staff there by making enquiries while I jumped the barriers and boarded the next train to Edinburgh, where I would start a new life as a bohemian poet wearing many scarves.

My real misadventures were less dramatic, and mostly devised with my new friend. Jemma was tiny, dark-haired, and seemed younger than she was. She sat in a corner of the girls' lounge, hunched and silent, worrying furiously. I made it my mission to divert her and make her laugh, with surprising and gratifying success. I had, by some means, got hold of the self-titled debut album of Christian country singer Amy Grant, recorded in Nashville, Tennessee, in 1977. There's a track called 'Grape, Grape Joy' in which the teenage Grant sings:

Don't give up hope, ye heavy laden.
You don't want to be a raisin!

I played the CD for Jemma, and we were breathless with laughter, lying across my bed.

'I mean, it's so true,' she mused. 'I *don't* want to be a raisin.' After that, whenever one of us was glum, the other would offer, 'You don't want to be a raisin,' as consolation. Imagine our delight at snack time when there were little boxes of raisins.

One afternoon, on my way back from the on-site school to the residential building, I managed to evade the nurse who was chaperoning us. I dashed off the path and around the corner to the window of the room where, if my calculations were correct, Jemma would be seated in a one-to-one with the psychiatrist. We called him Dr Pinhead.*

My prediction was bang on the money. I couldn't have asked for a better set-up: Dr Pinhead had his back to the window, while Jemma was facing me. Her eyes gleamed

---

* For legal reasons, I have been advised not to describe him, but you might imagine what a man called Pinhead might have looked like, hypothetically.

with recognition and surprise, but she kept her gaze steady. I pressed the button on an imaginary lift and slowly bent my knees, glancing at an imaginary wristwatch on the way down. Her lips twitched. I was attempting the stairs mime when I stumbled and lost balance, quite accidentally, but the result was total slapstick, funnier than anything I could have done on purpose.

In one moment, Jemma burst out laughing and Pinhead turned around. I dropped to the ground and held my breath. Nothing happened for a really long time. As I lay with my face in the gravel, it occurred to me that I hadn't thought this through. I snaked painfully along on my elbows, past the window. Somehow I got away with that one.

Another time, Jemma and I persuaded all the other girls sleeping upstairs to bring their duvets into the corridor, and we had a midnight feast – like a madhouse Enid Blyton parody – with snacks I'd stolen from the kitchen, knowing full well that the pegs wouldn't want snacks, so more snacks for me. Jem and I sang 'Grape, Grape Joy' in our best country and western style. A cowboy hat was fetched from somewhere. I brought out my CD player and a smuggled copy of P!nk's seminal album *M!ssundaztood* – originally confiscated for the one song in which, once, she says 'fuck'. We played that song quietly and took turns to be on watch by the stairs. I'd memorised the schedule for staff to patrol at night and every eighteen minutes we all dashed back to bed, bundling away the food and CD player and everything else.

I had one other great friend and ally at Maplewood, and that was one of the nurses. They weren't all unpleasant or unreasonable. Some were kind. Still, Giddy was unlike the rest, indeed unlike anyone I'd ever met. He was a practising Druid, for one thing, a sort of Green Man figure. He used to sit around strumming his guitar and singing songs that he'd written. There was one about the Conservative Party that went, 'Hey! You! If you'll be the colour of blue, there's a whole lotta Sheriff of Nottingham but not a lotta Robin Hood in you . . .' Predictably, I adored him. I counted down the hours until he was on shift; the whole feel of the place changed.

I had a nemesis, too. Harriet's hair was dyed black and so straight it looked as if she dipped it in ink. She was dripping alternative culture, from the chains hanging off her wide-leg jeans to the flames up the sides of her trainers. We fought like cats in an alley, and it was all because I loved and admired her desperately. Harriet was *cool*, and everything she did was cool because she did it. I was not cool, and she noticed that, and I hated her for it.

Harriet never thought anything: she *knew* it, and from experience too – and she could always tell you why what you had assumed, in your naivety, was completely wrong. Although we had both just turned fifteen, she put me to shame, she was so worldly. She'd had sex. She'd taken drugs. She spoke of such things in a casual, off-hand manner. She arrived at Maplewood a few weeks after I did, with the sense that she was just passing, dropping in from an adult world of people like her, a world about which I knew less than nothing. If she would only consider me her equal, I'd be content to be locked up in this purgatory of perpetual bollocking for the rest of my life. But, alas, she did not, and there was no reason for her to conceal how totally underwhelmed she was by everything I said and did.

When it transpired that we were both fans of Soundgarden, I was admitted, briefly, to the hallowed space of Harriet's bedroom. It was decked in posters of bearded, scruffy men standing about moodily. I stared at the moody men in awe. I was buying time by talking about the hospital's four-week assessment process before a diagnosis and treatment plan were decided upon.

'Oh, they've already diagnosed me,' she said. 'A long time ago. I'm bipolar. That's why I take lithium.'

I hoped I might be bipolar when they got around to deciding. It's rock-solid, I thought, you can't argue with it. A high-quality mental illness.

I excused myself to the loo and sprinted along the corridor to Jemma's room. I stuck my head around the door.

'Pssst, Jem!' I hissed. 'What is Soundgarden? I told Harriet I like Soundgarden, because she likes Soundgarden, but I've never bloody heard of it!'

Jemma shrugged, and opened her mouth to speak, but I was already marching back to Harriet, entering the room a little gingerly this time.

'Who's that, then?' I asked, nodding to one of the band posters.

'That's Soundgarden.'

'Oh! Oh, yeah. Of course it is.'

I made a pantomime of wiping my glasses on my sleeve.

'You're ridiculous,' said Harriet. 'Get out.'

I crossed the corridor again, back to Jemma's room, and landed heavily on her bed.

'Did you find out what a sound garden is?'

'Oh, yeah,' I said dully. 'I'm a huge fan.'

My own four-week assessment period extended to five weeks. I never knew why. It was to culminate in a 'professionals' meeting', which was, in fact, a series of meetings in succession. Every YP went through these, and a full morning or afternoon was set aside. They involved various combinations of your named nurse, your parents, and all the high-ranking people you didn't see very often: consultant psychiatrists and psychologists, various others you may or may not have met before. They would all discuss you, and some parts you were permitted to hear but for others you would have to wait outside. For some parts, your parents were allowed in and for others they had to wait outside. Such meetings were held monthly for the duration of your stay.

I was so ready for this. A proper diagnosis, not speculation this time, but informed by five weeks of round-the-clock observation. A bespoke treatment programme. It had been a long and difficult road to get here, and finally, it was all going to make sense. They were going to explain why I hurt so intensely and intolerably such a lot of the time. There would be a plan to make it all better. In time, and with the right help, I wouldn't need to self-harm for temporary relief, and I wouldn't crave permanent relief either. I didn't want to die. I wanted to live, but to do that I needed to not be in so much pain. This was the beginning of the end of that pain, and of the horrible clinging-on. I was ready to weep with relief, and the professionals' meeting hadn't even started yet.

The big day was a Friday. Meetings were happening elsewhere – meetings about me – and I was in the girls' lounge, all buzz and static and nervous energy. I could see I was driving everyone spare, hopping around, cracking

jokes, playing solo Bop It, but I just couldn't help myself.*
We all exhaled together when, finally, I was called into a
one-to-one with Dr Pinhead.

As I stepped into the small room – outside which, a
week or two earlier, I'd embarked on my physical comedy
career – I thought I might burst with fear and excitement.
I might just splatter all over that window.

'So,' he began. 'You've been here for five weeks now—'

'I know.' I realised as I spoke that I was interrupting
him. 'Sorry. I was just wondering: have you decided what's
wrong with me yet?'

'Well . . .' He hesitated. 'I would say that you're moderately depressed.'

'Only moderately? I've been in hospital for over a
month.'

I couldn't keep the disappointment out of my voice. It
wasn't that I *wanted* to be seriously mentally ill, but after all
this . . . it had to be something more. Moderately depressed
just didn't explain what needed explaining. And I'd been
taking various depression tablets for nearly two years. They
did fuck-all. An abyss started to open beneath my feet.

'But I would say that the main issue is an emerging borderline personality disorder.'

'What do you mean?'

'We use the word "emerging" because you're under
eighteen. A personality disorder diagnosis can't be confirmed until you're an adult.'

---

* Bop It is a rather noisy game which is played by following a series of com-
mands issued by a hand-held device: pressing the button, pulling the handle,
twisting the crank, spinning the wheel, and flicking the switch. The instructions get faster and faster.

'Oh. So, what's the treatment for that?'

'Personality disorders don't typically respond to treatment. This is just the way you are. You can go home next week.'

———

Later that afternoon I sat beside my parents in a crowded room full of adults. Some of them were strangers. Some I had met once or twice. They were seated around a huge table, and in front of each was a small stack of paper. They were all looking at me. I was afraid for a moment I had committed some ghastly crime that I couldn't recall.

Pinhead delivered the verdict. There was to be no further treatment. I was to be discharged in a week's time, back to 'care in the community'. But there was no care in the community. I knew that, and so did my parents, and so, presumably, did everyone around that table.

To my surprise, Mum spoke up. 'But what should we do?' she asked. 'If she's suicidal or if we think she's going to hurt herself, what should we do?'

Pinhead looked irritated.

'Well, if you're *really* worried, take her to A & E.'

'What will you do, though?' Mum persisted. 'Will you take her back?'

'No,' he replied firmly. 'She's being discharged.'

I had to get away – away from Dr Pinhead, away from all those eyes on me, away from Mum and Dad, away away away. As soon as I was permitted to leave, I ran through the residential building, past the hatch where they doled out our meds, past the wall where we queued for them, around the corner . . . As I passed the girls' lounge, I hollered, 'I'm going home!' in a tone that might have been celebration rather than despair. I leapt up the stairs two at a time and didn't stop running until I'd thrown open the door of my hospital bedroom and slammed it behind me.

I stood, panting, with my back against the door, and frantically surveyed the room. My cherished CD player was on the floor beneath the window, along with a small stack of my CDs. The paper inserts printed with lyrics were all out of their cases and scattered around untidily. My *Moulin Rouge!* poster hung above the bed. Jane Hunt was lying on my pillow. Her mismatched button eyes stared, unseeing.

I hurled myself onto the carpet at the foot of the bed and curled up into a tight ball, my eyes squeezed shut.

The thoughts that were mine and not mine came in rapid succession. I heard Pinhead's voice all over again.

This is just the way you are.

A personality disorder.

You can't be reached. You can't be helped.

You will always be this way and feel this way because it is who you are.

This suffering – your own and what you inflict on your parents and everyone around you – will only end when you die.

After a while, Jemma came and rested her chin on my shoulder.

'You don't want to be a raisin.'

A folded piece of paper slid under the door. Jem fetched it and handed it to me. It was a letter, written in silver gel pen on deep-purple letter paper, and it was signed at the bottom – from Harriet.

I read the letter quickly. Harriet had heard I was going home. Did I want to bury the hatchet and be friends?

I did want that. Harriet was still hovering in the

corridor, and we buried the hatchet then and there. We buried that hatchet so deep. On my last day she gave me her battered copy of Elizabeth Wurtzel's memoir, *Prozac Nation*.

'*Please love it as much as I have,*' she wrote inside the cover. '*It will be there in your darkest moments.*'

—

I almost can't believe I was at Maplewood for only six weeks. It felt like a lifetime. Were the doctors, and many of the nurses, really as cruel as I remember? I'm not sure. I don't know what they said to me, only what I heard. And I know that I left that place more hopeless, more suicidal, more demonstrably mad than when I arrived. I'd gone in willingly, confessing my every thought and waving reams of poetry at whatever poor sod was assigned to me that day. This was met with some bemusement, and I was often in the shit for various minor offences, but it had never occurred to me that the whole ordeal could be for nothing. They assessed me at great length and found me lacking, or undeserving of whatever it was that they offered.

As soon as I was home, I fantasised constantly about going back, being readmitted, and doing it right this time. I would understand how to be good, and they would see that I wanted to get better. I would be there a few more months while I had treatment, and then I would come out again and everything would be okay. I couldn't make it happen, so I did the next best thing: I daydreamed it, and I dreamed it at night too. I had a recurring dream that I was on a sofa in the girls' lounge, and that the top layers of my skin had turned flaky and transparent like dead skin, or dried glue. I was peeling the layers off, one by one.

I had a 'leaving book' – still have it, in fact. Once discharge from Maplewood had been arranged, the person who was going chose a notebook and left it in the girls' lounge for everyone to write a parting message. I was astonished by the warmth of the comments and wishes contained within my own, even from those with whom I'd not always been on the warmest terms.

'*I've enjoyed getting to know you,*' wrote my named nurse. '*We've had some interesting discussions and you've challenged me at times . . .*'

'*You are the most bestest best friend that I have ever had before in my whole entire life . . .*' began Jemma.

Harriet was more reserved: '*I know we have not been the best of friends in our time here, but I do care . . .*'

My favourite page was Giddy's. He wrote:

> *Cultivate the Wild Woman within you,*
> *yet do not become the Wild Woman.*
> *That way you will burn your brightest*
> *without exploding*
> *and a star such as you will sparkle on*
> *in this lucky world.*

I framed it and put it on my bedroom wall.

The Genius Disease

I seek forever the right way to know this.
That there are bridges
not built in me. That there are areas
that do not light up—

Bianca Stone, 'Reading a Science
Article on the Airplane to JFK'[1]

Autumn and winter 2003

I didn't see another psychiatrist or mental health nurse for months after I left Maplewood. I didn't go back to school. Mrs Wentworth was still holding off on her threat to expel me on the condition that I co-operate fully with all psychiatric treatment as prescribed. My place was kept open, but I couldn't face it, and no one was inclined to force me to go. I spent most of my time on the computer, at a desk beside the dining table in the middle of my parents' knocked-through downstairs rooms. When everyone was out, I scoured the internet for information about borderline personality disorder, or BPD as it was called. I pasted everything I could find into Microsoft Word and highlighted all the bits that sounded like me.

I was caught between dread at the words 'personality disorder' and relief at any framework I could hold up like a mirror and see something that was, if not actually me, at least recognisable. There were lengthy articles which explained the characteristics, thought processes, and behaviour of people with BPD. I thought that if I read enough of them, I might understand myself better. I might yet begin to see a way to be different.

Eventually I was sent to the Child and Adolescent Mental Health Service (CAMHS) in a converted Victorian villa across town: threadbare brown carpet, magnolia walls speckled with leftover Blu Tack, and leaflets everywhere. There were leaflets in piles on every surface and leaflets in transparent plastic leaflet-holders mounted on the walls. They had titles like 'Are you worried a child may have an eating disorder?' and 'Know the facts about drugs' and, most alarming of all, 'SEX: ANY QUESTIONS?' The radio in the waiting room played the same five chart toppers on a loop.

The psychiatrist there was Dr Anderson – or 'Pamela' as I never called him out loud – next in the line of oldish men to assess and drug and reassess me. He prescribed a new antipsychotic for what Dr Pinhead had rather dismissively termed my 'overactive imagination'. It was becoming more and more of a problem. I would hear my name called in the distance, whispering in the wardrobe. I couldn't shake the sense that someone, somewhere, was watching me and taking detailed notes. I told myself not to be stupid, but it was as if voices were beamed on radio signal into the inside of my skull: *You're doing this on purpose. You're inventing problems for yourself. You're attention-seeking.*

It didn't feel like my imagination. My imagination wasn't frightening. My imagination was respite from everything else that was frightening. I'd developed a lingering unease that nudged me to retrospectively analyse every interaction with other people, grinding teeth over every word I'd said, conjuring all sorts of disapproval and contempt. Had I said the wrong thing? Had I been inappropriate? There seemed no way to tell. I was frightened of everyone, frightened of being frightened, and frightened of how ridiculous that was. The new meds made my head feel like it was stuffed with cotton wool. In the evenings, my legs would twitch of their own accord.

I collected my prescriptions from the GP surgery, where I attended appointments in between seeing the psychiatrist. The waiting room had slippery chairs, a green speckled carpet, and low tables stacked with copies of *The People's Friend*. I read the soppy stories to distract myself and thought that I would like to write stories for a magazine – one day, when I grew up. If I grew up. I was beginning to doubt I'd make it that far. My own stories were not the cheeriest and it was probably just as well that nobody read them.

As she printed off my prescription, Dr Sawyer told me that I needed to be more positive. I should write a mantra – something like 'I'm going to get better' – and repeat that over and over to myself whenever I felt 'low'. She spoke with such easy confidence, as if she knew all about feeling 'low' and it was quite simple to fix. But whenever I felt anything – whether low, high, in the middle, or five miles diagonally and round a corner – I couldn't recall ever feeling anything else. The idea of feeling any other way seemed utterly absurd. I considered trying to explain this to Dr Sawyer, but I was always trying to explain, always talking and never heard, and I was losing appetite for it. So, I said, 'Thanks. I'll try that.' Dr Sawyer smiled approvingly.

I managed to peek at her computer so I could see notes and correspondence about me, the juicy stuff that wasn't sent in the post. Craning my neck, I saw two 'working' diagnoses – just as well, I thought: if you're going to have a diagnosis, you want it to pull its weight – 'Depression NOS' and 'Occasional Bulimia'. Not a whiff of personality disorder. I dashed home and went straight to the computer, sat impatiently through the shrieking of the modem, and asked the internet. NOS stood for Not Otherwise Specified: it meant I was depressed but in an unspecific way. Even the internet didn't know how I could have bulimia just occasionally. That there had been no mention of personality disorders was a relief, but unsettling at the same time.

There were a dozen regular doctors at the GP surgery, as well as locum doctors who visited from time to time. Each took a different approach to monitoring my mental state. I didn't mind Dr Sawyer, but Dr Quinn scared the ever-living fuck out of me. He was always slightly out of breath, and his sweaty palms left damp tracks on his trouser legs. His lips were moist, almost Barbie-pink. He smelt faintly sour. The patient's chair was positioned right up close to his, and I had to concentrate to make sure that my knees didn't touch his knees.

Dr Quinn reminded me of a Goosebumps book about a librarian who is secretly a monster with a huge swollen head and bulging eyes. The monster eats flies when no one is looking. At one point he eats a turtle. Dr Quinn definitely ate flies and turtles and god knows what else in between appointments. There must have been a tank full of turtles in that cupboard behind him, their scaly little feet moving hopelessly against the glass.

Dr Quinn asked a lot of questions. Were the meds working? Yes. Any problems? No.

It was uncomfortable to sit sideways, pointing my knees away from him and towards the cupboard full of turtles. I had an ache above my hip.

He continued, 'And you haven't had thoughts of harming yourself in any way?'

There was a pause as I mentally counted the cuts quietly healing on my thighs and upper arms. I recalled the debate I'd had with myself less than an hour earlier about whether I could get away with necking the leftover tablets in one go, whether it would do me any actual harm, whether there was any point. The only thing I really knew for sure was that if this was going to be my life, I did not want to live it.

I could hear Dr Quinn's quick, shallow breaths. Why did he breathe like that?

A dull thud from the cupboard. It shook ever so slightly.

I stifled a small, scared laugh.

I said, 'Nope!' a little too loudly. And I was free to go.

'*I want to stab him,*' I wrote in my diary when I got home, '*and throw him in a big bin.*' In retrospect this does seem a little harsh.

—

Perhaps the new meds were helping. I couldn't decide. I still felt like shit but, after all, it was impossible to know how I'd feel in a parallel universe where I wasn't taking them. Maybe I'd feel even worse.

I went back to school for Year 11 and managed to keep myself on the hamster wheel, although I was measurably stupider than I had been. Maths baffled me for the first time in my life. '*Laura has lost a little of the edge,*' my maths teacher wrote at the end of term, '*that made her such a strong candidate in Year 9.*' She was right: my mind felt like a blunted instrument. I got a B in the mock GCSE exam and was horrified. In hindsight, it's funny, how I threw up my hands, but I've never been pretty, or outgoing, or good at singing or drawing or sports. Being clever was all that I had.

I felt madder than ever, but I wasn't acting particularly mad. The chasm between what happened inside me and what happened on the outside stretched wider and wider. What my body was doing and saying, what everybody saw, was so far removed from everything I was feeling and thinking. Who was to say which was reality? If I dropped myself from one of the manor-house turrets, if the ground slammed into me, could it knock me back into myself? I craved the full force of impact, head to toes – *whoomph*, it would go, and I would be an integrated being. I would curl up into a ball, cry, scream, throw things. Instead, it was as if my body was programmed to steer itself around, talking to people, doing homework, eating jacket potatoes at lunch ... It was a sort of marvel, and it was desperately lonely.

Harriet came out of Maplewood and almost immediately went back in somewhere else. There was a shortage of beds, so they sent her to a private hospital, known as a 'Priory' – like where celebrities go after they party too hard. She wrote that the food was delicious. We exchanged long letters in scented gel pens, always careful to number the pages so they didn't get shuffled out of order. She sealed her envelopes with a red sticker shaped like kissing lips. I opened them carefully, sliding the nail of my smallest finger inside, and felt those mists of lostness and longing rise inside me. It was a feeling I could almost touch, like a tongue on a tooth.

I wanted to go back into hospital so that I could do it right this time, be believed and understood and guided out of this labyrinth that only ever seemed to go deeper. What was the secret that Harriet knew, and Jemma, and the others who were allowed to stay out their treatment? There must be a knack to making people see. If I could only turn myself inside out, render visible the blood and guts and anguish, they would know that I was indeed very mad and that I wanted and needed that intensive help. Instead, I stayed at school, behind my own peculiar force field of pain, cutting myself at every opportunity and writing endless stories and poems and diaries. I was haemorrhaging words, but there were never enough words to bridge that yawning divide within me, or between me and everyone else.

Dr Anderson was pleased with my progress. 'If you carry on like this, I'll be out of a job!' he quipped. I smiled and mentally called him a slimy git. He was so pleased, in fact, that he gave me a new diagnosis: bipolar disorder. Just like Harriet. I couldn't wait to write and tell her. Dr Anderson said that my recent improvement in functioning, namely going back to school, showed that I had 'responded' to the latest drug he'd added to the antidepressant and antipsychotic I was already taking. This new drug was called sodium valproate. It was known as a 'mood stabiliser' – as if I were moving through the world on the emotional equivalent of a wobbly bicycle.

They were big purple pills, like horse pills, and they made me bigger too. Stretch marks had appeared on my hips and thighs. When I pointed out that weight gain wasn't helping my mood, Dr Anderson replied, 'You don't strike me as the type to be vain.' He said that the fact that I was back at school proved that I was at least somewhat better, and the fact that the mood stabiliser had prompted this proved that the problem had been bipolar disorder all along.

Dr Anderson explained that my brain was wired incorrectly. It was an imbalance of chemistry. An invisible defect. Nobody's fault. I was born that way, prone to wild and unpredictable changes of mood. There was no cure, but so long as I always took my medication and followed the advice of my doctors, I might lead – well, not a normal life, but a life. 'A *relatively* normal life,' he said. This was on the condition that I did as I was told. Any future happiness depended on my taking all these pills every day without forgetting, and I must submit to medical advice because my own thoughts and ideas were not always to be trusted.

So, this was it. This was why it hurt to breathe, why I was so angry, so desperate, so terrified so much of the time. Why every emotion carried me along like a tidal wave, wrecking everything in my path. Why I caused my mum and dad and everyone around me so much grief. Why everything and nothing was wrong all at once. Why I just couldn't handle the day-to-day, the business of being alive.

Bipolar disorder explained everything. Not just all the misery, but all the not-misery in between. It explained how excited I got, how caught up and preoccupied, whether that was over my writing or a particular book or idea. It explained those times when I let my imagination take over and arrange the universe around me like my own dolls' house. I paced round and round my parents' dining-room table with music on, chattering away to myself, gesticulating, inhabiting a world that was however I wished it. This was crazy behaviour. *Manic* behaviour.

And it explained those times when I had too many thoughts at once and they all branched off like a family tree, each breeding half a dozen more, endlessly growing and multiplying all over the place. I spoke faster and faster then, but it was no good: I could only say one thing at a time, while all the other thoughts were there, waiting impatiently for their turn, still spawning wildly, unspoken. That was called *flight of ideas*. I loved that phrase – as if my ideas had stepped back to take a run up, sprinting along with deter-mined little faces, gradually lifting off the ground, legs going round and round in circles as they wobbled and gained height, until they soared rapturously into the clouds. All these peculiarities and more were known collectively as *hypomania* – another addition to my personal lexicon. It was so handy to have all these new names for things.

My meds came pre-packaged, like a gift. I took them home in a green paper bag from Lloyds chemist and unwrapped the little white cardboard boxes. On each was a sticker printed with my name and date of birth, and, inside, the shining silver blister packs. Sometimes I jabbed the pills from the back with my index finger so that they burst through the foil with a satisfying popping sound. Sometimes I slid my fingernail around the pill outline and carefully peeled back the button-sized silver sheet. It was like an Advent calendar that went on for ever. I wrapped my diagnosis around me, a warm coat. It was a reason. It was someone to be.

Dr Anderson spoke of the many famous historical figures believed to have been afflicted with bipolar disorder – great artists and writers and thinkers. Geniuses. Vincent van Gogh was the example he gave. The only two things I knew about Vincent van Gogh were: one, that he was a painter (sunflowers, starry swirly sky), and two, that he cut off his own ear. I hoped I wouldn't ever cut off one of my ears. My glasses would dangle off my face. Once I tried to put in contact lenses and I burst a blood vessel in my eye. I imagined myself staggering about with one ear and bloodshot eyes, blinking furiously and bumping into things.

I searched online for 'famous people with bipolar disorder' and it seemed to be quite literally all of them. This was cheering. There were multiple webpages listing these gifted individuals, and they included many of my own heroes, like Sylvia Plath. I was obsessed with Sylvia Plath. It's a little embarrassing to admit – not because Plath herself is embarrassing, but because it's such a cliché. I used to carry a battered copy of her collected poems around with me in my bag so I could revisit one or two whenever I was alone. Several other writers I admired had also made the list, having been diagnosed either during their lifetimes or posthumously (the latter hardly seems credible but at fifteen I didn't question it). Virginia Woolf was one. They tended to be women. Some lists helpfully noted cause of death beside name and occupation, and I couldn't help noticing that almost all these people had, sooner or later, ended their own lives.

Biographies assured me that these women were doomed

from the start. They were not for this world. Being talented and being mad and being destined for a violent, untimely death – these things were so tangled in one another that it was hopeless to prise them apart. It was a dangerous seed that Dr Anderson had planted, and that these lazy biographers watered. Did anyone think that mythologised, romanticised, fetishised, or just plain stupid accounts of dead women writers might have consequences, not just for their families, but for impressionable, literary-minded girls questing to find out who they are? It would be too awful, I thought, to be mad and then dead and to not even leave some good sentences behind. My writing took on new urgency. It became essential that I publish something really spectacular before my inevitable early demise.

Was it inevitable? As I pondered my diagnosis, I was unsettled by its permanence: a lifelong condition. It spoke not just to who I was at fifteen, but who I would be all along the span of my life. That life was still a mystery, an endless series of plausible alternatives arranged into a giant question mark. I wanted to travel, have adventures, meet brilliant people, fall in love, dive head first into all human experience . . . Instead, I faced a lifetime of trying this drug and that drug, seeing this doctor and that doctor, probably in and out of hospital. It didn't seem like much of a life. Perhaps I would kill myself, or perhaps something would eventually work. I'd hit on a particular combination of tablets that would make things radically easier, but then what? I wanted to go to university but had missed so much school I could only be entered to sit half my GCSEs. It seemed unlikely that any university would let me in. I wanted to get married, one day, and have my own children. It seemed even less likely that anyone would want to marry me.

I've always wanted to be a mum, ever since I was a little girl myself. I never gave much thought as to why. It just felt right. It was a part of me that was sleeping until the time for it to wake, just as I had put my baby dolls to sleep in their wooden cots, tucking their little blankets around them. I tried on motherhood the way I tried on Nan's cocktail dresses – in play, to see how it felt. Around the same time, I had a pale lemon-yellow smocked party frock I inherited from one of Mum's cousins. I longed to wear it, but it was far too big. It hung in the wardrobe, and I liked to look up at it and rub the hem between my fingers. Then, one day, it fitted me. I wore that dress on my sixth birthday, and it felt just lovely. Similarly, I had always expected to grow into being a mother.

I asked Dr Anderson what my bipolar disorder meant for my having children – 'Not now, obviously,' I added hurriedly, as his eyes widened in alarm, 'but one day. I've always known that I wanted to have children one day.'

He told me that he wouldn't advise it. He said that there was a grave risk of my becoming very seriously unwell after having a baby, and I could never be sure of the stability I'd need to be an effective parent. Also, bipolar disorder is genetic, which meant that I could pass it on. The chances were as high as one in four.

That was when I decided not to contemplate the years, perhaps decades, ahead. I would take one day at a time, and travel hopefully. There was always a next thing to try: a new medication, a counsellor or therapist, another diagnosis, book, diet, religion, whatever. Maybe I would never be completely better – I couldn't imagine being better and still being me – but better was, after all, comparative. Maybe I could still be bipolar, and it didn't have to hurt like this. Maybe I could still have a future that was defined by something else.

I was holding out for a miracle, even a rescuer – a psychiatrist, therapist, teacher, healer; I didn't care who it was or, really, how they did it, but someone must have the answer to how I could stop feeling like this. That's not to say I planned to sit around passively while someone else fixed everything for me, although I wouldn't have minded that if it was going. I was willing to do whatever it took, but first I needed to know what that was, and I was clueless. There had to be a hint hidden somewhere in the universe. The alternative, that there was no answer, and I would always be this way, was unthinkable. If I allowed that spectre of suggestion to creep in, I was on a bridge, on a balcony, beside a railway line, ready to jump within minutes.

And so I remained at sea, caught between competing narratives of my own distress. On one hand, there was nothing wrong with me besides a general tendency towards silliness and attention-seeking. I still saw Mrs Wentworth in assembly at least once a week, standing at a lectern on the stage of the school hall and rattling off her pet slogans. 'Happiness is a choice,' she stated. But on the other hand, I had been born with a terrible disease that required medication and monitoring for the rest of my life. Dr Anderson was quite certain of that. I had my answer, finally, and it only spawned more questions. What did this diagnosis mean? What was chemistry and what was character? Where did bipolar end and I begin?

two

Rota Fortunae

Inconstancy is my very essence; it is the game I never cease to play as I turn my wheel in its ever-changing circle, filled with joy as I bring the top to the bottom and the bottom to the top. Yes, rise up on my wheel if you like, but don't count it an injury when by the same token you begin to fall, as the rules of the game will require.

Boethius, *The Consolation of Philosophy*[1]

Summer 2010

'Beams!' I exclaimed, charging into the cottage. The letting agent shuffled in the doorway as I enthused about the dark, rather battered-looking beams in the ceiling, and Jon quietly accustomed himself to our new home. It had been built around 1750 as part of a larger house, which was then divided up into a series of two-up, two-down workers' cottages, with a toilet and shower eventually tacked onto the back. It was painted in standard rental-property magnolia with the standard cheap beige carpet, but it was old, and I was already in love.

'Just look at the fireplace!' It was massive. I climbed in

and twirled with my arms out, my fingertips grazing the brick – until it occurred to me that there were probably spiders in there. I stepped out quickly, tripping over the edge of the hearth.

We moved in a few weeks later with a hired van driven by my dad, and some friends to help us lift and carry. As we sat on the floor among the boxes, eating our takeaway pizza, Jon mused that he would never have pictured this as his adult life, in an eighteenth-century cottage with me. He seemed happy. He set up all his computers and gadgets, wires trailing around the edge of every room. I arranged my books on the shelves alphabetically by author's surname. Month by month, we bought some furniture.

Our previous home, advertised as a maisonette, had come with its own furniture. We were skint, newly married, when we'd moved in the year before. It was a new build in a terrace that was off the main road, facing a petrol station, and the walls were so insubstantial we could hear the neighbours sneezing and going for a piss. It was a bit like the channel that used to show a twenty-four-hour live broadcast of the *Big Brother* house – except, of course, that we had also unwittingly signed up to be on *Big Brother*. Any conversation we didn't want overheard had to be conducted in whispers, and our sex life was timed carefully around when both sets of next-door neighbours would be out. The neighbours had no such qualms. One day the curtain rail in the living room crashed down spectacularly onto Jon's head, and for this the landlord had the temerity to blame him. We called it the Cardboard House, and we were not altogether unhappy when it was sold from underneath us and we had to move.

The new house, or the new–old house, was as solid as

houses come. Not only that, but there was a pub a few doors up the hill: a good pub, with window seats, an open fireplace, a garden, and beers that Jon said were decently kept. (I wouldn't know, because I drank rum and Coke in those days.) It was neither a trendy pub nor an old-man pub, but a place where students and locals rubbed shoulders, and everyone knew everyone else. It became our home from home. I had discovered alcohol as a sort of social lubricant: the way it convinces you that you're enjoying yourself; its warm, convivial glow. There were long Sunday afternoons playing board games, and late-night lock-ins until the German landlady came downstairs in her dressing gown and told us all to fuck off home.

Despite being quite consistently mad, I'd finished some GCSEs and A levels – although with worse grades than predicted – and off I went to my second choice of university. From there, with sympathetic lecturers and extensions to essay deadlines, I came away with a first-class degree in English and Classics, only to immediately dive back in for a one-year master's in Medieval Studies. Jon and I were married that summer, and he moved from London to settle with me in a small university town in Surrey. I had planned to write about medieval literature, but I got sidetracked and ended up researching and writing a biography of a fifteenth-century vowess.*

I was addicted to the thrill of finding stuff out. It fired off all the reward centres in my brain, the ultimate dopamine hit, and I would gladly trawl through documents for months in pursuit. How bone-achingly cool to be the first person to read something – to know something, however

---

* A vowess was a woman who took a vow of chastity without becoming a nun.

inconsequential – in half a millennium, to rediscover what we have collectively forgotten. It was those crumbling Elizabethan steps at school all over again: a hand reaching out through the centuries, a glimpse of another world where everything and nothing is different.

Long days in the windowless manuscripts room at the National Archives paid off. In fact, they culminated in a full-on victory dance, to the bemusement of everyone present, when I found a few words in a preface to a series of deeds that conclusively proved my hunch as fact. I wrote up my MA dissertation rapidly and gleefully, then felt bereft. The only solution was to start a Ph.D. on vowesses. Others had caught my eye and were waiting in the wings.

One was Margaret Beaufort, mother of Henry VII. He was her only child and she dedicated much of her life to putting him on the throne, despite his dubious claim. It was reported that, at his coronation, when 'her son was crowned in all that great triumph and glory, she wept marvellously'. She had been through hell and back for this – at one point narrowly escaping execution for plotting against Richard III – but she wasn't weeping for joy. She was weeping because 'she never yet was in that prosperity but, the greater it was, the more always she dreaded the adversity'.[2] I knew the feeling.

This was the Rota Fortunae, Wheel of Fortune, an ancient idea that was popular at the time and lingers now. Just as night becomes day and day becomes night, as the moon rotates through her phases and the seasons through summer and winter, so our own personal circumstances revolve in a circuit of good times and bad. If you hit rock-bottom, the only way is up. If you're on top of the world, you had better brace yourself. What goes up must come down.

Bipolar was my Wheel of Fortune. Once bestowed, the diagnosis became a part of my self – as much as my thick curly hair with its tinge of the ginge, my bookishness, my asthma, my perpetual nervousness about potential spiders . . . any of the traits and quirks and characteristics that jumble together into who we are. At the same time, bipolar was bigger, more fundamental than anything else. The noun and the adjective were one and the same. I was asthmatic, but I was not asthma. I *was* bipolar. It wasn't so much a case of living with it as living around it. There were days when it took centre stage and swelled and bloated there, expanding outwards until it consumed everything, and on those days managing it was a full-time job. But not every day was like that. I was thankful to have my studies, my friends, my husband and our little rented cottage, all this in spite of everything.

I took all my tablets meticulously, the big purple mood stabiliser and the antidepressant and antipsychotic. I kept the blister packs on top of the kettle where I would see them when making tea in the morning. As I swallowed them down, I shuddered to think what I'd be without these little daily micro-doses of sanity. The weight gain, sleepiness, and other side effects were an encumbrance, but I put up with them as gracefully as I could, and I was never late to an appointment.

There were such a lot of appointments: the psychiatrist, my allocated mental health nurse, the GP, the university's disability service, my support worker. There was always someone to whom I had to report. I briefed every lecturer who taught me in advance. In fact, I briefed almost everyone I met. 'If my behaviour is strange, this is why. If I'm dragged screaming out of the room by men in white coats, this is why. Thanks for your patience.' I made a lot of jokes. They weren't very funny.

My university psychiatrist was unlike any psychiatrist I had met before. Dr Radcliffe was a woman, for one thing. She was about my mum's age. There was something owl-like about her, warm and feathery. Her eyes were slightly magnified by her glasses and her navy-blue eyeliner. She came from the local mental health service to the health centre on campus, and we had long conversations about bipolar disorder. She answered my endless stream of questions about what it meant and what my life would be. These were hour-long appointments, sometimes every week, a luxury I doubt anyone is afforded now. Her view of my situation was more optimistic than Dr Anderson's had been: bipolar may not be curable, but, with the right meds and the right support, I could live well alongside it.

One day I nervously raised the question of having children, expecting Dr Radcliffe to echo what Dr Anderson had said years before. What to him might have been a passing comment on something too distant to be relevant was already etched into my psyche. His verdict bothered me, in part because I could never wholly accept nor reject it. Just as I'd hurried to reassure him that I wasn't planning a pregnancy at fifteen, I got that disclaimer in quickly when I broached the subject with Dr Radcliffe, but now I was twenty-two and had been married over a year. Jon and I weren't about to start a family just yet, but it was a glimmer on the horizon.

I mentioned that we had talked about having children – 'not now, obviously, but one day' – and quickly followed up with, 'But I know I might not be able to have children – or, rather, maybe I shouldn't – because of my bipolar.' I tried to make it sound like an afterthought. I didn't want to admit to having set my heart on this.

In fact, Jon and I had talked about children, in an abstract future tense, even when I was an undergraduate and he was living in a house-share at the shitty end of Greenwich with no wardrobe and no proper bed. We were lying, wrapped up in each other on the mattress on the floor, surrounded by his clothes and bits of computer, when I asked him if he wanted to have children one day. Although it was still impossibly distant, and perhaps distantly impossible, children were a dealbreaker for me. I was so relieved when he answered yes, without hesitation.

Dr Radcliffe didn't hesitate either. 'Of course you can have children if you want to,' she said. 'You'll be a lovely mum. I mean, yes, there is a risk attached to it, but we'll have a plan and keep a close eye on you.'

There were many follow-up conversations. What did she mean by a plan? What would that look like? How likely was it that I'd go fully batshit after having a baby? Could I take my meds if I were pregnant? How likely were any children to be bipolar as well: was it really one in four? Did that mean that, hypothetically, if I had three children, and each of them was a one in four, that's three in twelve, so still one in four? Surely if you have multiple children, it becomes more likely . . .? I'd never liked statistics. It was all very well doing the maths, but this was my actual life. Potentially someone else's actual life.

Dr Radcliffe would let me run out of questions, take a breath, and answer each of them in turn. This was interrupted by further questions, and some questions got lost along the way. She sketched it out for me: 'I'll get the call that you've delivered, and I'll be straight down to that hospital for my baby cuddles and to see how you are.'

I could see it so clearly – not so much Dr Radcliffe visiting me on the maternity ward, as nice as that would be, but a baby in my arms. My baby. Mine and Jon's baby.

It never happened, at least not like that. Dr Radcliffe took early retirement and was gone. How could she? I thought, unreasonably. After all, I was used to doctors and nurses and whoever else ricocheting off my life. I met someone once or twice or twelve times, discussed things that were intensely personal in a forced, artificial way, and never heard from them again. Rinse and repeat. I was well trained in detachment – not so much detachment from other people as detachment from myself. I stated the facts of my own life as if speaking about someone else. But Dr Radcliffe was different. Somewhere, during the five years or so that I knew her, the dividing line between the me who lived my life and the me who reported on my life had slipped. When she disappeared, as they all disappear, it was a sort of grief. I don't remember saying goodbye.

Dr Radcliffe's replacement was Dr Freyman. He didn't come to campus, so I had to get two buses to see him in a run-down building on the site of the local hospital, about six miles away. Dr Freyman was a grey-haired, grey-suited man – more of a Dr Greyman, really – and similar to Dr Anderson in both appearance and outlook. Once again, I was not so much a person as a collection of symptoms. I stopped thinking so much about babies after that.

Titanium

. . . for we all of us, grave or light, get our thoughts entangled
in metaphors, and act fatally on the strength of them.
George Eliot, *Middlemarch*[1]

Autumn and winter 2012–13

I was face down on a floor that moved like the ocean,
surging, awash with the shattered fragments of a mil-
lion shells and bones and fossils. My mouth was open as
if I were calling for help, but I was not calling for help.
My lungs were empty, the breath knocked right out of
me. Above, the cold glare of the ceiling lights rendered
everything overexposed, like a washed-out photograph.
Everything buzzed and fizzed. There was no getting
away from that relentless light, no scrap of comfort
anywhere.

I was in the bin – and by 'the bin' I mean a psychiatric
ward. I call it that not to be edgy or to make a joke of it,
although gallows humour has served me well enough, but
because that was what it was like: a rubbish bin for human
beings. The people there had given up on life, and, worse, life

had given up on them. They sat blankly on stained armchairs in front of daytime television.

The nurses were indifferent at best and violent at worst. They emerged from their little locked 'station' only when there was a ruckus of some kind, in which case they would rugby tackle the offender and then fuck off again. If you said or did anything they didn't like, they had a habit of leaping on you, throwing you onto the floor, and pinning you there while they injected you in the bum with sedatives. That was how I came to be flattened, right by the door, which was three inches thick and the only way in or out.

Afterwards, when the drug wore off and I stopped bumping into things, I was more careful of what I said.

It had been almost a decade since I was at Maplewood, and for all my nervousness about future mental health crises – or 'episodes' as they were known – at some point I had edited out the possibility of going into hospital. This was the price of my complacency. As if psychiatric hospitals assemble themselves around people who aren't paying attention and can only be kept at bay through constant vigilance. Never forget, I told myself. Never forget this can happen to you at any time. Even when things are going well, you're just on the other side of that door.

What scared me most was that I couldn't remember how I had come to be there in the first place. I had wanted to die. I had planned to die. Had there been an attempt? I wasn't sure.

Retracing my steps, it was clear things hadn't been going so well. My Ph.D. felt like groping in the dark, and I'd found myself doing anything rather than research – or, more accurately, doing nothing rather than research. I suddenly forgot all my Latin. This unnerved me because I didn't understand why it had happened, but also it was a very real impediment to reading documents that I needed to read. I hid in the pub instead. I didn't want to be at home because I couldn't face cleaning the house, and the uncleaned house bothered me. The cottage had a problem with damp, and I found that our board games had gone mouldy in the inbuilt cupboards. I felt mouldy: morose and dark and dank – a dripping, rotting dungeon of a person.

I decided to sort it out. I scrubbed the kitchen floor. I put all the board-game pieces in ziplocked freezer bags. I began memorising the noun and verb endings I had learned when I was twelve and used regularly ever since, and I gritted my teeth against the fact that it was as if I'd never seen them before. With Dr Freyman's permission, I also started gradually, tentatively reducing the dose of my aripiprazole. Aripiprazole is not, as I first thought, the name of a character in *Good Omens*, Terry Pratchett and Neil Gaiman's fantasy-comedy masterpiece, but an antipsychotic drug. My hope was that, if I took less of it, I would be less stupid and sleepy and fat, but also ideally no madder than my baseline acceptable level of madness.

I lost a stone in three weeks, and I was thrilled but I couldn't sit still. Everything itched. Colours were brighter, sounds were louder … the whole world was aflame with possibility, if only I could settle to something. This culminated in a sort of waking dream that a friend of mine, who had died a couple of years before, was trying to contact me from beyond the grave. I agonised and theorised about how to help her. At one point, I boiled my meds on the stove.

Jon was suitably alarmed and phoned my care co-ordinator, the nurse assigned to me at the mental health service. Her name was Annette. She wasn't there. Jon left a series of messages with a series of receptionists. Annette eventually called back and offered an appointment in two weeks' time. The best she could do, she said.

And then somehow, I was in the bin, relieved to have finally found the toilets but less relieved to note that I had my period. I rummaged in my bag, knowing full well I hadn't brought anything. Then I knocked on the door of the nurses' station and stammeringly asked a male nurse if they had any tampons or sanitary towels. He chuckled and said, 'No, we don't do that.' I improvised with loo roll and hoped for the best, then continued to explore my surroundings.

It was a mixed-sex ward with two ten-bed dormitories. Each bed had stiffly pleated blue hospital curtains you could pull around. There was also a large room with straight-backed armchairs arranged around the perimeter and a television in one corner, and what was ostensibly a games room but which only had various components of different games: a Scrabble board but no tiles, around a third of a jigsaw puzzle, and a huge table-tennis table with no balls or bats. I don't think anyone was raring for a game of table tennis, but it was like they'd put it there to make a point.

Later that afternoon, we were herded downstairs to a canteen where custard was the colour of highlighter pens. It glowed faintly, as if radioactive. Beside the canteen was a paved courtyard, but it was overgrown with weeds and we were not allowed to use it.

Bedtime came around and I discovered that zopiclone – the sleeping tablet I was prescribed from the age of eleven or so, until I became rather too fond of it – was handed out to everyone with their night-time meds. Small mercies. I popped my pills and climbed into bed, wriggling under the thin sheet and blanket tucked into the sides, like a human pitta bread. I lay back, with my papery curtains pulled around me and a jumper over my face to block out the light, and I dropped into oblivion, suddenly, like falling off a precipice.

I couldn't breathe. My jumper was blocking my nose and mouth. And it was heavy, smooth . . . My jumper was not a jumper. It was a pillow, and it was being pressed down over my face.

I flailed and gasped and pillow filled my mouth, cotton sticking to my tongue. I heard a muffled yell in the distance. My fingers buried themselves deep and my arms thrust forward. The pillow came away easily, flying sideways towards the door, where the blue curtain around my bed had been pulled aside. Two glassy eyes met my own, staring in the sunken face of a grey, wraith-like figure of a woman. The figure was staggering backwards from the force of my shove, staggering with the ragged, shaking steps of a corpse. Its eyes were locked into mine.

The ward was haunted by a vengeful, murdering ghost.

The murder-ghost was wearing pink flannel pyjamas, which seemed somewhat out of character. I recognised her then as the woman who slept in the bed opposite. She had ignored me when I'd said hi on my arrival some hours earlier and ignored me again when I'd called over 'good night'. I hadn't thought much of it at the time, but I remembered with my heart still hammering in my ears, and I thought, How dare you not be a ghost, how dare you be an ordinary mad person and frighten me like this, how dare you try to smother me in my sleep after I said hi to you earlier.

'What the fuck?!'

She stood mute and expressionless. Then, she gathered up her pillow from the floor, held it to her chest, and stated, solemnly, 'I'm going to kill for Simon.'

'That,' I spat, 'is the creepiest fucking thing I have ever heard.'

She turned wordlessly and went back to her cubicle, where she sat upright, entirely still, and she watched me.

I clambered shakily out of bed and rearranged my curtain. I could feel her eyes boring into it, and through it, into me.

I decided to stay awake that night. It seemed the safest course, and I thought it would be easy enough, with an aspiring assassin in the bed opposite. But as I arranged the sheet and blanket over my legs again, I could already feel tides of sleep tugging at me, dragging me down to the depths. I forced my eyes open, imagining my eyelids pinned to their sockets, but I must have dozed because I jolted and gasped and tasted pillow and faced those staring, shining eyes all over again.

'I'm going to kill for Simon.'

It was as if I was trapped in a nightmare, stuck on a loop that wouldn't end. As if she really was a ghost, suspended in time, reliving the same scene over and over. I was part of it, this strange dance, the two of us entwined. What were we enacting? What had happened? What was about to happen?

Nothing was about to happen, I resolved firmly. I disentangled my legs from the sheet again and glared at my assailant. She stood in the same spot, clutching her pillow to her chest as before.

'I'm not having this,' I announced to no one in particular.

'Shut up,' came a groan from the bed next to mine.

I pushed my weight against the heavy door of the dormitory and stepped out into the corridor. It was deserted, the floor cold and gleaming under my bare feet. Even my breath seemed to echo, my still-banging heart reverberating endlessly as I made my way to the nurses' station.

The door had a small square of clouded Perspex and I tapped on it. On reflection, I was keen to remain alive, ideally for as long as possible. If I did die – when I did die – I was certainly not going to be murdered by Skeletor in pink pyjamas.

The door opened several inches and a head emerged.

'What?'

'It's the woman in the bed opposite mine.'

'Uh huh?' There was a note of irritation in the nurse's voice.

'She, erm, keeps trying to put a pillow over my face when I'm asleep,' I said.

The head was retreating back.

'Could you help? Please?'

The nurse sighed, opened the door a few inches further, and squeezed herself through the gap. She gestured behind me. Skeletor had followed and was standing in the corridor, facing the wall of the dormitory.

She stepped back from it a few paces, took a run up, and flung herself at that wall as hard as she could. The impact was loud, and it knocked her to the floor. Immediately she picked herself up and did the same thing again. Over and over. It was as if she was expecting Platform 9¾, and every time she staggered to her feet, she looked a little more dishevelled, a little more desperate.

I turned to the nurse and tried to read the expression in her eyes.

'She's very poorly,' she shrugged, and as I began, 'Aren't you going to—' she closed the door in my face. It swooshed as it shut and clicked decisively.

This was a holding pen, I realised. Nothing more. No one was going to help us in here.

Scuffs and smudges were appearing on the wall, like when a bird flies into a window.

As I heard the woman's face smack into that wall again, the clatter of teeth, I wanted to do something for her. I wanted her to be able to rest. I wanted the sound to stop.

'Hey,' I called to her. 'Hey!'

She didn't seem to hear me. She heaved herself to her feet again and started to shuffle backwards, eyeing the wall with wary determination. I braced myself.

I was sorry that I'd called her Skeletor, if only in my head. She was very poorly. She didn't know what she was doing. If it was understandable for any compassion I might have felt to be diluted by her repeated attempts to murder me, still I regretted it. Here was a human being and she was unwell and vulnerable, and she should have been looked after, her dignity protected. I shouldn't have called her Skeletor.

Crunch. She hit the wall again, and a small smear of blood appeared, trailing down to where she lay in a crumpled heap. I crouched beside her. She was panting, her eyes half open.

'Can I help you back to bed?'

She didn't respond.

I crouched there uselessly for a while, afraid to touch her, then went back to my own bed. It was on the other side of that wall, so that we were both lying down – me on the bed, her on the floor – with the wall between us. I dreaded hearing her body slam into it again, but there was only silence.

The silence was worse. I found my jumper under the bed and put it on over my nightie. I gathered up my phone and the novel I knew I wouldn't be able to read, and I took them to where she had been. I could sit beside her, at least.

She was gone. There was no trace that she had been there, or that she had ever existed, no trace except the bloodied scuffs on the wall.

She wasn't in the lounge or the games room or any-where else that I could see. The ward was empty, the nurses tucked away in their little locked room, the patients in their dormitories lost in deep, drugged sleep. A muted peace had settled over the place like resignation to despair. I stood in the games room, alone in the half-dark. Then I went to the window and looked out.

The psychiatric inpatient unit was on the same hospital site as the clinic where I saw Dr Freyman. There was also a large building with general wards, a maternity wing, and innumerable other buildings, some as small as huts or bungalows, with no identifiable purpose. Twisting paths connected all these destinations, and dotted around were car parks, grassy verges, a tree or a bench here and there. From the first-floor window, I couldn't see much except rows of parked cars, but in my mind, I soared above, and I could see everything. I scanned the hospital complex and, beyond it, the town and the world that were still out there. All those people sleeping in their own beds, or lying awake, and none of them knew we were here.

I ignored the zopiclone tugging at my arms and legs and eyelids, urging me to lie down, and I searched for the moon in the sky. The moon stared back with a hard gaze. Its indifference was oddly comforting. It existed millions of years before I did, and it would still be up there long after I was dead. Almost everyone in human history had seen that moon. It connected us all, across thousands of years and thousands of miles. In that moment, the moon would be visible to Jon, if he looked for it, and visible to everyone I loved and everyone I would love but hadn't met yet.

'Back to bed!' came a gruff voice from the nurses' station.

As I trudged along the corridor to the dormitory, a thought occurred to me: I hadn't been sectioned. I was a voluntary patient. I could go home in the morning. I had consented to go into hospital because the doctor at A & E had made it clear that I was going in whether I consented or not. A voluntary admission meant less paperwork for him, and probably a shorter stay for me: win-win. Once these bizarre negotiations had been concluded, I was bundled into the back of an ambulance, and . . . there was lost time there, but it didn't matter. I would tell them tomorrow that I was leaving.

The woman who wasn't Skeletor never came back. I didn't find out where they had taken her, or why. She simply vanished. I began to wonder if I'd dreamed her. Maybe she really had been a ghost. I reminded myself not to entertain thoughts like that. That was how you ended up in the bin. Or perhaps what landed you there was believing your eyes and ears, trusting your own impressions over what you were told.

The nurses wouldn't let me go home, nor would they tell me why I wasn't allowed to leave. That was how I got flattened.

—

On every psychiatric ward I've known, the radio was a permanent feature, so that whatever was in the charts became a soundtrack to that admission. Sometimes, even now, I hear one of those songs in a café or a pub and it transports me back. Then I go and stand outside with the smokers or walk off down the road, just because I can.

Maybe it wasn't the radio. Maybe they only had one CD. Either way, 'Titanium' by David Guetta and Sia blared out of that nurses' station over and over and over. The synths made my gut clench, and in my mind's eye I saw an endless line of chomping, grinding gears. As a madhouse anthem, I had to admit it was perfect. I mouthed along my own rejection of flesh and blood, a declaration that I was invulnerable, unable to be knocked to the ground. After the flattening, I wanted that more than ever before. I would have sold my humanity for it in a heartbeat.

Instead, I seemed to disappear. I never did it consciously or even knew that it was happening, but more and more often I would reach for a memory and grasp at nothing, a trail of smoke. Where did I go, in the absent times?

Time moved differently on the ward. It was sluggish, constipated, as if the air itself was on a truckload of meds. I watched clocks and paced around each room, up and down each corridor in turn, counting the minutes and hours and days. If not pacing, I was trying to get mobile signal so I could contact the outside world, squashing myself against the games-room window and holding my phone as high as I could reach until my arm ached too much to continue. I was allowed to keep my phone but not my charger. Probably just as well, I conceded, as I would probably have been garrotted with it that first night, but preserving battery was a constant concern. The only way to charge my phone was to hand it in to the nurses, but then it could be a long while before I managed to get it back.

I didn't tell my family where I was. I reasoned they had suffered enough. As had I. It was bad enough being there without worrying about how other people might be feeling about my being there. If I could have kept it a secret from Jon, I would have. I did feel a twat, though, squeezed against that locked window and on the phone to my mum, pretending everything was fine.

'Not much happening here,' I said, watching a man being hauled out of an ambulance and into the building. 'It's all been pretty quiet.'

The problem with lying is that once you start, you have to keep it up. Self-harm taught me that, and it taught me to be convincing as well. I'm a terrific liar. Not my most endearing attribute, but there it is.

Once a week, half a dozen of us were collected from the ward and taken to 'art therapy'. We were led through the building to a room in which a box of craft supplies had been tipped over a large table. The craft supplies were mostly bits of coloured card. A nurse stood guard in the corner, but aside from that, we were left to our own devices. I knew there would be no scissors, but I checked anyway. Then I rummaged grimly among the Pritt Sticks for one that had retained its lid and was still sticky, and I undertook a similar exercise with felt-tip pens. With the three working felt-tips I'd found, I made a birthday card for no one in particular, then dropped it into the waste-paper basket on my way out.

The same suspects had 'talking therapy' in another room, where plastic classroom chairs had been arranged in a circle. No one wanted to talk. I spent the allotted forty-five minutes mentally mapping the ground floor of the building, or the parts of it I'd seen, and I tried to calculate how I might get hold of a lanyard that would let me through the doors. Every scenario I played out in my mind ended with my being seized and sedated almost immediately, unless I had a gun or had become very suddenly adept at kung fu. Even if I did get out, where would I go?

To my surprise, Annette, the care co-ordinator who had been too busy to see me, came to visit the ward. She escorted me to a small room with flaking yellow paint and a framed print of a vase of flowers, a room more depressing because someone, a decade ago, had made a half-hearted attempt at making it not depressing. There was a great crack along one wall.

'How are you doing?' she asked.

I raised my eyebrows and gestured around myself.

Annette scooped her blond hair behind her ear and clasped her hands in her lap in a manufactured-empathy pose. 'I know,' she said. 'It's such a shame.'

I looked away stonily. The printed flowers were so unflowerlike. The crack in the wall seemed to have grown, spreading and reaching, ivy over a ruin. It occurred to me that the roof might collapse. The hospital could implode and swallow us all like a dying star. It was a shame all right.

I said as little to Annette as I could get away with. Too late, I thought.

I did have more welcome visitors. I was the only patient who did. I was thankful: it's not easy or pleasant to go inside a psychiatric hospital to spend time with someone. Jon came every few days and said very little. He looked tired. Our friends from the pub, god love them, turned up nervously in twos and threes. Friends from other places came too, and not always the people I expected. They brought me little gifts: useful things like toiletries, and useless, loving things like CDs I couldn't play but would keep for ever.

Nicole brought me a brick of a fantasy novel – her favourite, on loan. It should have been such a treat. The ability to stare at a dead tree and hallucinate vividly for hours on end has been one of the great joys of my life. It's an escape, a rest, a forgetting – a small holiday from being myself. But when I needed that most of all, the letters blended and merged, rearranged themselves, ran like inky spiders over the page. Somewhere in this episode, this breakdown, this such-a-shame, I had lost the ability to read. I willed myself to trust that it would come back with time, as would my Latin, as would everything. I slept with the book under my pillow. I took it out at night and held it to my face.

From the window, I saw Nick arriving with half a dozen board games stacked precariously on his bicycle. These included Hotel, which is like Monopoly but with planning permission; UR: Royal Game of Sumer, reproduced from a game found in the ruins of the ancient city of Ur, Mesopotamia, and dated to approximately 2500 BCE; and my favourite, By Jove. It's based on Greek mythology and has a stack of oracle cards printed with things like: 'The FATES, who control mortal lives, find you without any redeeming social values, so go to HADES!'

I had no one to play board games with, but that didn't matter. In this place where no one ever had fun, here was proof that fun still existed. I held my games and books and CDs in my hands, and I knew that I would take them home with me. There would be a time after this time. How odd it was to go into a place ostensibly to receive care, and then for all the care to come in from outside. The care signed a visitors' book and was escorted on and off the premises.

The only way out of the bin was to be discharged, so my mission became to persuade the hospital psychiatrist that I was fit for release. It was his call. I nodded eagerly as he stated that the reason for this relapse was the recent reduction in my aripiprazole. This meant that he could put the dose back up, and up a bit further for good measure, and the problem would go away – the problem being me, and away being home. I played my part beautifully. I took the drugs, kept my head down, and each week I told the psychiatrist that I was feeling better – but not so much better that it wasn't believable.

I made a suitably convincing recovery and was discharged, only to be readmitted soon after and have to do the whole dance again. I found that getting out of hospital was one thing but getting the hospital out of me was quite another. The surroundings had soaked in: the smell, the stiff curtains around the bed, the weird glittery floor, the echoing. It was all there when I closed my eyes.

Two admissions – or was it three? – in under six months. In, out, in, out, this bizarre hokey-cokey. Once there were no beds available and I was sent to a different hospital. That was much nicer: you could help yourself to drinks whenever you felt like it, and converse with the other patients in a comradely mad-person fashion. I was devastated when a bed became free at my local and they shunted me back.

The hospital psychiatrist put me on lithium. This came with a perpetual parched feeling, the need to piss every half hour, and a slight hand tremor that was a disconcerting reminder of Nan. My hands became her hands on the day she put down her knitting and never picked it up again, the first time she handed me a biro to fill in her crossword. It stank of decline. I went out of hospital on day release and drank pints of orange squash to flush the lithium out of myself.

I couldn't tell you precisely when any of this was, or in what order it happened. If I try to establish the chronology or locate events that are missing, my brain pops up an error message. Access denied. There's probably a password somewhere, but I'm not going to rummage too hard. I don't mind admitting that I'd rather not know.

Later, the Care Quality Commission would deem that psychiatric unit 'not suitable for modern mental healthcare' which is a bit like awarding Castle Dracula one star on Tripadvisor. It was so stark, so hopeless, so ridiculous – the embodiment of the state of mind that had landed me there in the first place. It was as if depression were a physical space that you had to go and live in every time you were depressed, or as if someone had created an immersive art exhibit to represent how depression feels. It was far removed from the cosy surroundings of Maplewood, but I don't think I was as shocked as I might have been – or as

I am now, remembering. I don't think it occurred to me that I deserved better.

At the bottom of the wheel, I could only try to cling on tight and trust that it would pass. It did pass. The visits and gifts kept me in touch with the world enough that I could persevere. I'm not sure that lithium did much to hasten better days. More than anything, it seemed to be just the passage of time. With a great creak, my wheel lurched upwards as daffodils were breaking out on the banks around the hospital grounds.

I went home. I bought posh custard from M&S at the petrol station, and I ate it from the plastic pot with a teaspoon, chilled and creamy-sweet. I went to the pub, and we played By Jove in the garden until evening drew in, then settled beside the fire. Nicole's husband, Ramsay, scrawled *ALLOWED OUT* on a beer-pump label and made it into a badge for me. We stayed late that night, long after closing. I spaced out my rum and Cokes with soft drinks because of the lithium, and I didn't mind too much.

They were always like this, these mood swings of mine. Whenever I felt one way – good or bad – I could never remember anything else. It was a blessing as well as a curse, this forgetting. Almost on purpose, I took those weeks and months in the bin, and I shut them off from myself. They became only facts – toothless, colourless. I banished all those nightmare images to a distant land, and I planted my flag in the soil of life and hope and normality.

An Act of Infinite Optimism

When it comes to you, when it just happens easily, it is still the biggest gamble in the world. It is the glorious life force . . . what's meant to be – but really to create a human being is a huge thing. It's huge and scary – it's an act of infinite optimism.

Gilda Radner, *It's Always Something*[1]

Summer 2013

In the weeks and months that followed my release, I integrated back into ordinary life with surprising ease. It was as if I'd never been away. My spell in hospital became a blip, an aberration, a bad dream. Sometimes I doubted it had happened at all. Then one day I found myself at the sink beside the toilet at the back of our little rented cottage, and in my hand was a positive pregnancy test. I stood there in my nightie and gaped at those two unequivocal blue lines.

I didn't know what to do with myself, with the news. I paced up and down, round and round the house, the cheap beige carpet rough between my toes. I should tell Jon first and I should tell him in person, of course, but he had gone to work, and he wouldn't be home for another twelve hours. What would I do for twelve hours?

I put the kettle on. While it was boiling, I remembered that there's caffeine in tea. Was I allowed tea? Would it hurt the baby? The baby. Oh god. Better not.

I sat at my desk upstairs and picked up a microfilm printout of a fifteenth-century will I was halfway through transcribing. I stared at it blankly. Nope. Absolutely no way.

I watched the clock for ten minutes. Tick tock. *Fuck it.* I called Jon.

'Yeah?' There was background noise.

'Jon ... I'm ... I'm ...'

'What?'

'I'm pregnant. With a baby. An actual human baby. We're going to have a baby!'

'I can't talk now. I'm on the train.'

'What? Seriously?'

'It's packed. People will be annoyed.'

'I don't care! Jon, I'm pregnant!'

'I know. I'll call you when I get in.'

'People will be annoyed,' I muttered, hanging up.

Counting on my fingers, it had been fourteen days since we'd planned this in the pub over my final rum and Coke. It seemed ludicrous, suddenly, to just decide to have a baby one evening and then go home and, ahem. Was it ludicrous? My mental health was much better. Jon and I were settled. We could afford it. Children had always been part of the plan. My Ph.D. funding rather miraculously included maternity pay, and who knew when I would get that again. We wanted several children eventually, probably, and not all in nappies at once, so best not leave it too late. We weren't ready – god, no – but is anyone ever actually ready?

It wasn't supposed to happen straight away like this. The morning after the pub conversation, I'd bought pre-conception vitamins from Boots and read the entire internet on the subject. That was quite something. I'd spoken to a few people I knew who had babies. All the evidence suggested, really very strongly suggested, that it takes ages to get pregnant. The more reputable websites assured me that the average couple takes six to twelve months to conceive, and because I was fat, we were looking at longer than that, perhaps significantly longer. I anticipated doctors' appointments and fertility tests and lots and lots of waiting. I was settling myself into this new life phase of trying to conceive. Except, of course, that I was already pregnant.

Jon called back: 'I figured you'd be just as pregnant when I got off the train.'

'I do seem to be. How are you feeling about it?'

He thought for a moment. 'Daunted but pleased.'

'Yeah, same.'

We both said 'wow' a lot. There wasn't much else to say. We would go to the GP and find out how to access midwifery care. We'd need to move to a bigger house.

I phoned my mum next. 'That was quick,' she said.

I wanted very much to tell my friends. All of them. In fact, I wanted to tell the whole world this momentous news. I wanted to paint it on the side of a building. I wanted a megaphone. But there's an unwritten law that you're supposed to keep pregnancy a secret until after the twelve-week scan at least. I felt myself bumping up against another of these strange social rules upon which I hadn't been properly briefed. It was presumably in case of a miscarriage, but if something that awful happened, I would want my friends to know so that they could support me. What was I supposed to do – tell them I had been secretly pregnant but wasn't any longer? In which case, why not tell them now? It seemed absurd, the idea that I was supposed to grow a human for three months and just not mention it. It didn't seem possible. I told everyone.

I spent the rest of that morning pacing through the house, headphones on, harnessing the rhythm of music and the rhythm of walking to arrange my thoughts into some sort of order. I announced the news to myself over and over, each time hearing my own surprise. I bounced like a pinball between joy and worry, joy and worry. I did what I always do when I'm daunted by something, which is to reassure myself by daydreaming about it going extremely well. I saw a little boy, about five years old, with Jon's blue eyes and my curly hair. He could have been a girl, of course, but he didn't feel like a girl. I saw him in my mind's eye, and I loved him. I was going to do my absolute best for him.

I phoned the mental health service and left a message with the receptionist, half apologising: 'I just thought I'd better let Dr Freyman know.'

To my astonishment he called back, personally, less than two hours later. His voice sounded different over the phone. It was unsettling to encounter this disembodied version of Dr Freyman in my front room.

'We need to get you off lithium as soon as possible,' he said. There was a risk. Cardiac defects. The baby's heart.

'But I thought ... I mean, we talked about this before, and I thought—'

'Never mind what you thought,' he replied, his voice

uncharacteristically sharp. I heard him take a breath and adopt a measured, reassuring tone. The risk of heart damage from exposure to the lithium was around 10 per cent. The best thing to do would be to reduce the dose over the next few weeks and then stop taking it altogether.

But what about the aripiprazole? He said there was 'no known risk' in pregnancy.

'No known risk? Or no risk?' I didn't like pressing him like this, but it was important. 'Is there a known not-risk? Because I was told, with the aripiprazole and the lithium, it was okay and now apparently it isn't, and how am I supposed to get this right if it keeps changing all the time?'

I could hear that he was forcing himself to be patient. He explained that there were no published reports of harm to babies from aripiprazole but there was limited experience of prescribing it in pregnancy. I said I didn't want my baby to be the experiment. He urged the importance of keeping me stable. Another episode could be worse for the baby than taking the medication. It was a case of weighing up the risks and benefits, and, all things considered, I should taper down the lithium and come off it as quickly and safely as possible but continue to take the full dose of aripiprazole.

I'd been pregnant for five minutes and I'd already fucked it up. What had I been thinking? I couldn't keep house-plants alive.

Reluctantly, I agreed, and I was as good as my word, although I did cut down the lithium a bit quicker than instructed, and some days I half forgot to take my morning dose of aripiprazole ... Mostly, though, I did as I was told and kept swallowing my pills down, whispering apologies like a prayer.

Over the next few weeks, I was more tired than usual, and more tearful – 'changeable', as one of our pub friends put it, while I was frowning over my third lime and lemonade with everyone getting more and more lively around me. Thankfully I wasn't too sick, nothing a ginger nut couldn't sort out. I started carrying a packet in my handbag for emergencies. The pregnancy symptoms that bothered me most were the ones no one warned me about: nosebleeds, bleeding gums, an alarming new rash across my chest that I scurried off to get checked the moment it appeared. Pregnancy awoke my inner hypochondriac with a start, and I was constantly checking my body for signs, warnings, information. It was like reading tea leaves, except I was the tea leaves.

I knew it was a risky time, and that it would be wise not to get too attached to this baby – or, more accurately, to this embryo that I was hoping would become a baby – until that twelve-week milestone. I couldn't help it, though. The loss of this microscopic creature was already unthinkable. It was my speck of stardust, a spark of pure potential. How could I not root for it? The weeks crawled by maddeningly slowly, while I scuttled to the loo every five minutes to check I wasn't bleeding.

Finally, I hit that magic twelve-week mark and allowed myself to breathe, just a little. Everything happened at once, then. We were lucky to find a larger house, a proper family home, for not much more money in the next town a couple of miles away. We didn't realise, until we got the appointment letter, that the first scan had been booked for moving day.

Early that morning, I brushed my teeth with cardboard boxes piled around me and abruptly vomited into the sink. My parents were driving up from Southampton and collecting the hired van on the way. In a few short hours, I was in our new kitchen, unpacking the kettle and my decaffeinated teabags, and it was time to get back in the van and go to the hospital.

Sitting next to my dad, strangely high up and with the gearstick shuddering between us, reminded me of the blue van he drove when we still had the shop. Dad used to let me change gears for him. 'Second,' he would call, and I'd check the little numbers around the top of the stick to remind me in which direction to yank it. If I was out, he quickly adjusted it as he drove. Sometimes I rode in the back, standing on boxes so that I could 'surf' as we went round corners.

Soon I would be the mum instead of the daughter. My grandparents had been dead for years and the generations were shifting, everyone stepping up a place to make room for my baby.

———

'A strong heartbeat,' said the sonographer in a warm, confident voice. I was lying on my back, naked from the waist down while a sheet of something like oversized kitchen roll served as a nod to my dignity. She twirled a wand around inside me and abracadabra: an image appeared on the screen.

Craning my neck, I saw my son for the first time, kicking fierce little legs and sucking his thumb. I couldn't believe it. He was so very much a baby. Fuzzy-edged and large-headed, but definitely a baby. I didn't feel different enough to justify the fact that this human child was there, living and growing inside me. Evidently Jon was thinking along similar lines: he sat there with his mouth open, like a fish. We left with printouts of the scan images. I lined them up along the mantlepiece but found myself carrying them around the new house with me, so that I could look at them wherever I was.

A few days later, we had another appointment, this time to see the consultant obstetrician. Jon and I sat in the waiting area of the maternity wing of the hospital, sweating in the sticky August heat and surrounded by couples in various stages of pregnancy visibility, for a full hour and a half past our appointment time. It seemed maternity services were overstretched and underfunded much as mental health services were. Mostly I just wanted to know what the consultant would say about the baby's heart. When would we know if all was well?

Dr James was a brisk, capable older woman in a white coat. Extra scans were booked, including one with a specialist who would examine the baby's heart in two months' time. That would confirm – or, more likely, rule out – any damage from the lithium. All signs were good, Dr James assured us. And of course, there was a conversation about mental health. Dr James wanted to know about my family history. Had my mother suffered from any perinatal mental health problems?

Mum had told me about her postnatal depression more than once. After a long and difficult labour, she was about to be wheeled into theatre for a C-section when a Dr Denzel Elias – who was experienced in breech

deliveries and, the way Mum told it, quite possibly wearing a cape – intervened, and I was born just after 5 p.m. on
a wintry Saturday afternoon. Mum said that when she
held me for the first time, she felt a 'rush of love' unlike
anything she'd ever known.

In those days, it was usual to stay in hospital for up to a
week after the birth of your first baby, and up to two weeks
if you'd had a bad time. But as it was so near to Christmas,
we were discharged home when I was just a few days old.
Dad was running the shop and it was the busiest time of
the year: there was no question of his taking time off to be
with us. I cried constantly and, as often as not, Mum joined
in. Christmas and New Year passed in a blur.

Mum took me to our family GP for the six-week check-
up and sobbed in his consulting room. After that, the doctor
took it upon himself to turn up at our house unannounced
so he could see how Mum was doing. The health visitor
made extra visits. Nan and Auntie Pat helped a lot. As
summer approached, Mum's mood lifted, and she felt ready
to face the world again. That was the story I knew.

In fact, nearly all the women on my mum's side of the
family have had postnatal depression. One of my great-aunts
once confessed to me that, as a new mother in the fifties, she
kept all the windows locked in case she should be seized by
an inexplicable impulse to pick up her daughter and just
hurl her out. I was a little shocked when she told me that. I
couldn't imagine wanting to defenestrate my own baby –
except, of course, that it was the last thing in the world that
she wanted, otherwise she wouldn't have locked the windows. How horrible to be afraid of yourself like that, I
thought, to feel that you didn't know what you might do.

As I summarised all this for Dr James, it dawned on me

that I was pretty much guaranteed to go all sorts of mental in six months' time, if not sooner. It had been wildly irresponsible to get myself pregnant when it was so apparent that I wasn't up to it. Had I not already proved Dr Anderson right? I had bipolar disorder. I was mentally unstable, and impulsive to boot. And it wasn't just me who would be harmed. It was this baby, this new person. They could be scarred for life because of me.

Dr James wanted my assurance that, if I felt unwell postnatally, I would visit my GP. I said, 'Yes, of course.'

She filled in a form, and everyone was satisfied. The plan, it seemed, was that we would all cross our fingers and hope for the best.

So that was what we did. It wasn't too difficult, at least not most of the time, but I could never quite banish the worry. It was the spectre in the shadows. I felt okay — mostly, I felt good — but that spectre slumped ominously in corners of rooms, in my peripheral vision.

As the leaves started to turn, I unpacked the last of our belongings. Scans came and went, and all was well. My hunch had been correct: we were having a boy. We would name him Arthur. I carried the name with me like a talisman, always on the tip of my tongue. Arthur. I saw him again on the monitor, shifting and wriggling, almost dancing. When I felt him, it was not so much kicks as flutters, as if he were emerging from a cocoon. Something was beginning to awaken, to unfurl within me.

That pendulum swinging between love and worry, love and worry, found its centre and trembled there. The love and worry were one and the same, bound up in wonder. It's incredible how much you can love someone you've never met.

Rounding Apace

I'm a means, a stage, a cow in calf.
I've eaten a bag of green apples,
Boarded the train there's no getting off.

Sylvia Plath, 'Metaphors'[1]

Winter 2013–14

I had lost my midwife.

I established a routine of phoning the hospital every morning. Every morning I would explain that, yes, I'd had a midwife initially, but I asked to change to a different one because I kept turning up for my appointments and finding that she wasn't there, and it was stressing me out. So, yes, I'd spoken to the supervisor of midwives and, yes, I was assigned to a different midwife, but I had never met her or heard from her. I could see from the 'green book' of my maternity notes that antenatal appointments were overdue. I read out the name of my midwife from where it was scrawled in biro on the front page.

'Oh, she got married . . .'

'That's nice. Is she still around?'

'I'm not sure. Haven't seen her for a while.'

'Please could you find out?'

Every morning I was promised a call back that never came. I was seven and a half months gone and this daily pantomime was wearing me down. What could I do? Go to the hospital and camp out in the corridor until they put a blood-pressure cuff on me? Give up on antenatal care and just turn up when I'm in labour, assuming someone will assist? I was explaining the situation again one morning when the hopelessness of it struck me in a moment and I heard my voice crack.

'Don't worry.' The voice coming out of the phone was warm. It was a voice I hadn't heard before. 'I'll be your midwife. I'm Stella. When can I come and see you?'

Stella visited me at home every week after that. I saw her walking briskly from her parked car with a bag full of midwife kit, and on my way to open the front door, I thanked whatever benign force had sent her. There was something familiar about the way she wore her lipstick; she could have been any one of my aunties. I put the kettle on when she arrived, and we had proper conversations, not like those exercises in form-filling where I never held the pen.

With Stella in place, I could turn my attention to the two tasks ahead of me: first, to give birth safely and ideally with as little misery as possible, and then, to look after a baby.

What scared me about birth, more than anything else, was the prospect of going back into hospital. I shrank from the thought of those stiff, blue curtains surrounding me again. I started reading about home birth. Research suggested it was as safe as hospital birth, provided you were healthy and having a straightforward pregnancy. Two mid-wives would come to the house, and they wouldn't also be trying to look after a dozen other labouring women at the same time. I could have my own bed, my own pillows. No cubicle curtains or echoing corridors. Surely that would be better for my mental health.

I put this to Stella. My weight was a complicating factor: home births were 'not recommended' – which may or may not have translated to 'not allowed' – if you were over a certain BMI.* It seemed the same forces insisting I take medication that made me fat were relentlessly punishing me for being so: every time I saw a doctor it was brought up, or cited as the cause of whatever was ailing me; at every pregnancy scan it was lamented that my blubber was blocking the view. I read the research that the guidance was based on and made my counter-argument. I was active, on day-long hikes around Windsor Great Park well into pregnancy. I was generally healthy. The main concern was my psychiatric history, and my mental health was better served by birthing in my own space where I felt calmer and less crowded by bad memories. We would be close to the hospital if an emergency did arise. Stella listened to all this and filled in the home-birth form.

'They won't like it,' she said, 'but I'm with you on this one.'

Reading up on home birth, I came across the idea of a doula. A doula is someone who provides practical and emotional support before, during, and after a baby is born. I found yet more research papers which indicated that having a doula present at birth reduces the likelihood of

---

* Body mass index: a calculation based on weight and height, used to determine whether a person is considered to be a healthy weight.

needing medical intervention. Not only that, but it reduces the risk of postnatal depression. Here was another measure I could take. I couldn't control how the birth went, or how mad I went afterwards, but I was going to do everything I could to give us the best possible chance of the best possible beginning.

Jon raised his eyebrows at the cost. People spend thousands on their weddings, I argued. Surely this is as, if not more, important? Wouldn't it be great to have someone who could support us both, the same person throughout, someone who knew us and also knew about birth? An advocate, an encourager, an extra pair of hands? I emailed him all the research I'd read, and then emailed him a shortlist of local doulas with pros and cons of each. If only to empty his inbox, he agreed to meet a few of them.

'This doesn't mean we're having one,' he warned.

'Oh no,' I said. 'No, of course not.'

Lisa came to our house and sat in the armchair by the window with her little stack of doula paperwork. I knew the moment I saw her that she was the one. There's something about her that reminds me of sunshine, the gentle warmth of early spring. She didn't ask intrusive questions. She understood, without my needing to say it, that I was afraid. She understood that my strategy was to research the hell out of everything, and then implement what I'd learned with practical steps. In this, access to someone for whom being a birth nerd was a life's work was invaluable. We emailed back and forth. She visited again to do birth planning with us, talking us through the various options. I drafted a Word document and titled it 'Birth Preferences'.

—

It was time for antenatal classes. They were eye-wateringly expensive, but it would be worth it to be better prepared. I couldn't recall ever having changed a nappy in my life, and the prospect of either of us bathing a newborn sounded like a newspaper headline waiting to happen. We needed skills and knowledge, the practical stuff: Keeping a Baby Alive 101. The website also promised new friends, other families at a similar life stage with whom you could share teething anecdotes or something. I was less sold on this one. I didn't need new friends. I couldn't keep up with the friends I had. But I could see the value of mutual support that was specific to having babies, and I *was* beginning to feel a bit of an outlier, as the pregnant one.

On a rain-drenched evening in January, we approached the squat, red-brick building – half bungalow, half church hall – where we would meet the six other expectant couples for the first time. I gripped Jon's hand as we crossed the car park, dodging puddles that gleamed in the darkness.

'I don't want to do this,' I said very quietly as we passed through the doors.

It's not that I'm shy, exactly. It's just that I'd rather die in a fire than make small talk with strangers. Ever since I read about the Sorting Hat in 'Harry Potter', I've liked to imagine having a shouting hat. I would be there, politely nodding along to someone's inane remark with a forced smile on my face, lonely and uncomfortable and longing to escape, and my hat would suddenly announce, 'LAURA DOESN'T WANT TO TALK TO YOU!' at an astounding volume. I would apologise for my terribly rude hat – 'Hats, eh?' – but secretly I would love it, and I bet it would empty the room pretty quickly as well. What a relief.

Antenatal chit-chat consisted of a rapid exchange of information: due date, boy or girl, name choices, our careers, our ages. 'Oh, you're really young!' the other pregnant women kept saying to me. I had just turned twenty-six. What is the correct age to have a first baby? I wondered. Several of my cousins were still in their teens when they had their first. My mum had me at twenty-eight and her midwife described her as a 'geriatric' first-time mother. Everyone at our antenatal class was in their thirties. Steph was thirty-eight. I couldn't imagine being thirty-eight, but I restrained myself from saying so out loud.

During the tea break I hid in the sparse little kitchen, where there was a heavily limescaled kettle and boxes of herbal teas had been lined up in a row. It was freezing. The others had made their drinks and quickly taken them back to the main hall. I was rummaging through cupboards, looking for some normal tea, relieved to bury my face among the identical tiny mugs after forty-five minutes of 'getting to know you' time. I turned around and there was Hayley, all curly ginger hair and warm brown eyes and pregnant belly. We had met, but not really met, during Advanced Name Learning.

'Laura!' she said.

'Hi.'

'I love your necklace.'

'Oh. Thanks.'

It was a little silver teapot on a chain. My mum had bought it for my birthday a few weeks before. I flipped the catch so that it sprang open to reveal a tiny faux pearl.

'I love it! I bloody love tea. Do you want some tea? I'm spitting feathers here.'

We made tea. I clasped the mug in both hands, held it

up near my face to feel the steam. I didn't want to go back to the hall, not even for the electric heater.

Conversation turned to baby names. My choice of topic, just because I loved saying the name Arthur out loud. *Arthur.* Try it. It's lovely. Hayley duly admired it and said that she didn't know if she was having a boy or a girl, but if it was a boy, she would like to call him William, after her beloved stepdad, Bill, although she wasn't sure about that because his surname would be Grocock. She hesitated. 'I can't really get away with it, can I?'

'What, Willy Grocock?'

Whenever I want to laugh but I mustn't, I imagine dead puppies in a bag.

The bag sank slowly to the bottom of a dark pond.

I pursed my lips and tried to look thoughtful and diplomatic. There was silence.

I ventured, 'I guess you could home educate?'

Hayley laughed so suddenly and uproariously that I jumped, and then joined in, relieved. The mug had warmed my hands and the herbal tea wasn't too bad. Here, at least, was someone I could talk to.

'Bold move to take on the name Grocock, though. Or is that your original name?'

'No, my original name went on for weeks. Every time I filled in an application for a passport, I'd run out of little boxes for letters.'

Why are there so many penis-themed surnames, we wondered. You never hear any female equivalents. We started suggesting some.

Over the following weeks, Hayley and I swapped life histories. I had spent all my life at school, at university (arguably an extension of school), or in the bin. Meanwhile Hayley had been a DJ, calling herself Hayley Unlikely and living above a gay pub in London's West End. I didn't know there was such a thing as a gay pub. Were you only allowed in if you were gay? How would that be policed? Was there some sort of entrance exam? Were bisexual people allowed to loiter in the doorway? Even the notion of queer spaces was a long way in my future.

Hayley's house was full of vinyl records and rugs and ornamental owls. She had a hamster called Sid and spoke to him in a kind voice. Even nine months pregnant, she was whipping up a key lime pie in the evenings and crocheting gifts for everyone else's babies. She made dozens of car-seat blankets, trimmed with brightly coloured ribbon, each the size of a baby's lap with holes in the right places for the seatbelt and harness to go through. Talking to the others didn't feel quite so much like rubbing up against sandpaper when Hayley was nearby.

The more time I spent with other expectant mothers, the younger and more unqualified I felt. They all had established careers, while I was still a student with no idea of what I would do with my life except that I hoped it would involve being free to obsess about the distant past. Their husbands wore tasteful shirts, and I didn't understand what their jobs were. Business this and finance that and marketing the other. I supposed I wouldn't know what a web developer was if I hadn't watched Jon's fingers flying as reams of unintelligible code appeared on a monitor like a magic spell. I'd always liked his scruffiness; it was comfortable, leaning into his big hoodie, but he did look out of place among the other dads.

Gatherings were arranged in immaculate homes. Some had a shabby-chic vibe going on, and the other mothers-to-be clearly did a lot more hoovering than I ever have. I perched awkwardly on their beautiful cream sofas, thinking of the battered fake-leather one we inherited from my parents, and how it fell off its plastic feet if you moved it. I thought about the house I'd been so excited to move into a few months earlier, how everything was either a gift or second-hand, and none of it matched. Piles of miscellanea had a habit of appearing on surfaces. I was practically kicking aside copies of manuscripts and empty bottles of Captain Morgan. No way were they coming to ours.

While the women congregated in each other's houses and sat for hours, surrounded by fabric bunting, the men went out to the pub, or for curry.

'Can I be a man?' I complained to Hayley in an agitated whisper in somebody's gleaming kitchen. 'Where is my curry, please? It's bad enough that I haven't had a drink for nearly nine months. Last week I didn't sleep because I was chugging Gaviscon all night, and now Arthur's moved down, I think, and I don't sleep because I'm going for a wee every forty minutes. On the dot. They say curry is supposed to get labour going. It won't if it's the men who are eating it. I've heard that about pineapples as well. And sex, which is a joke. How's that supposed to work, pray tell? Jon can't get near me. I'm so massive I have my own gravitational pull. Small objects have started to orbit me. I'm going to order a curry when I get home. And naan bread.'

'Ooh, yeah, you should,' said Hayley. 'I've made a casserole. It's in the slow cooker. I know, it's a fucking nightmare—'

We were interrupted, again, and so it was back to trying

to ensure that my smile didn't look too much like a grimace.

We sat through long, lowering evenings and listened to talk of epidurals and forceps and ventouse and hypno-birthing, an array of options and scenarios. Lisa and I had already been through all this. I'd typed up my birth prefer-ences, and laminated copies were stored safely in several locations. Even so, as I listened to the rain battering the roof and windows, determined to break in and wash us all away, I was confronted with the idea of birth as if for the first time, the horrifying reality that I was soon to push an eight-pound screaming human out of my actual vagina. What the hell was that going to be like?

And what was I doing here, among these round, serene women, whose husbands were stroking their hands as they reflected on their birth choices and new lives ahead? They had their shit together, while I was winging it – my home, career, pregnancy, everything. That much was obvious, and no number of research papers or spreadsheets could com-pensate. I wanted so desperately to do this well for Arthur's sake, but I had a sickening feeling that I was not old enough, not wise enough, not middle-class enough, and, most of all, not sane enough to be his mother.

I was spared around half the antenatal sessions because they were exclusively about breastfeeding, which Dr Freyman had said was out of the question because of my meds. I asked the woman who led the classes if there would be any sessions about bottle-feeding. She said no. Instead, Lisa took me to Sainsbury's and gave me a tour of the baby aisle. We bought formula-milk powder, bottles, and a steriliser.

I went to my final appointment with Dr James, having prepped myself for another conversation about mental health. Surely we weren't just going to fill in that form. There must be something else we could do to prepare, or to mitigate . . . I was going to tell her about Stella, and Lisa, and antenatal classes. But when Jon and I were finally called out of the waiting area, Dr James wasn't there. Someone who worked for her discharged me from consultant care with a clean bill of very pregnant health.

Healthy I may have been, but I was larger and more uncomfortable by the minute. I took to our battered sofa and binge-watched a drama series about Sherlock Holmes, my feet propped up on cushions to bring down the swelling. Our cat, matronly and irritable in her oversized black cardigan, settled with me there. April had half a white moustache and a pleasing medley of pink and black toe beans, which under no circumstances was anyone permitted to touch. Resenting the lack of room on my lap, she contented herself with stretching out along my thigh, facing away to emphasise her displeasure at my inconvenient new body shape.

As another grisly yet intriguing murder case was solved, I flipped through *Mother & Baby* magazine. Endless photos of immaculately made-up women holding adorable babies. Nobody had sick on their clothes or looked dishevelled or exhausted or fed up. It was all a bit suspect, even to this ignorant reader who knew that the clock was ticking and her time of unknowing almost up. The pregnant women beamed and glowed, fingertips resting lightly on perfectly spherical baby bumps. Where were their swollen ankles? April had started licking mine, for reasons that were unclear, with her neat sandpaper tongue. I nudged her off and she flashed me a look of pure hate.

Admittedly *Cankles Monthly* would be unlikely to attract

many subscribers, and the idealised imagery couldn't be
that unrealistic, because the women from my antenatal class
wouldn't have looked out of place in this rag. They could
have had their own double-page spread. I could see, mapped
onto the pages, what their early weeks and months of
motherhood would look like. I couldn't see mine. Was
anyone in *Mother & Baby* bipolar? I guessed not. Somewhere, in the vast wide world, there must be another
pregnant woman as flawed and scared as I was.

—

My blood pressure began to leap up and immediately
duck back down again, like an elaborate prank. I would
attend routine appointments and find myself ordered
straight to hospital. I begged a lift off someone, got there,
was re-cuffed and then told to turn around and go home.
Lisa emailed me a list of Eleven Natural Ways to Keep
Your Blood Pressure Low. Then my heart started hammering like a demented woodpecker. Achy and breathless,
I returned to the maternity ward.

The heart monitor bleeped its alarm in a panicked sort
of way on and off, on and off, as hours went by. I closed
my eyes and felt myself drift. My eyelids were a night sky,
arched over babies in boats on an endless sea. I felt like a
boat myself, crossing unknown waters with this precious
cargo, willing the waves to be kind.

My reveries were interrupted by the arrival of a man
with a clipboard. He sat down beside the bed, introduced
himself as Eric, and said that he was a midwife. I must have
indicated surprise because he started talking about the difficulties of being a male midwife, how some women don't
want a male midwife, and isn't that sexist when you think

about it ... I wondered if there was a way to steer him on to what he had come to see me about. Presumably he hadn't dropped in for careers advice.

'Anyway,' he said, finally. 'We've noticed there's a home-birth form among your notes. I must tell you, we strongly advise you to come into hospital when labour starts.'

'You mean at four centimetres?'

I'd paid enough attention in antenatal classes to know that you're only considered to be in proper, hospital-going labour when your cervix is four centimetres dilated. What no one had explained is how you're supposed to be able to tell.

I eyed him doubtfully. 'I ... don't think I'll be able to check. I mean, it's really far up. I guess maybe if I had a torch, and a mirror? But I'm not convinced I'll be able to—'

'Oh no,' he laughed, gesturing with his hand to brush away the idea like crumbs off his lap. 'If you *think* you're four centimetres, you come in and we'll check.'

I hadn't the first idea how I'd estimate what my cervix was doing. This could cost me a fortune in taxis. Better not ask him to clarify further, I decided, so instead I asked if he was advising me to give birth in hospital because there was something wrong with my blood pressure or my heart.

'No, no,' he said. 'You're fine. We've run tests and every-thing's come back normal. You can go home as soon as you're ready.'

'So, why ...' I groped for words and gestured to the heart-rate monitor, then to the hospital bed I was lying on. 'Why is my heart rate so erratic?'

'Just one of those things, I suppose.'

What did that mean? Stella, when I asked her a few days

later, put it down to a combination of hormones and Arthur squashing me. He was squashing me *on the inside*, and I felt it too. Was it that? Was it because I was anxious? Perhaps, although I had experimented with concentrating very hard on my most distressing worries while attached to the heart monitor and that hadn't corresponded with numbers climbing or frantic beeping any more than resting had done.

'But come back if you have any problems,' continued Eric. 'And come back if you have chest pain, or a severe headache, or if you feel that baby is moving less, or if you're worried.'

Of course I was worried. Of course I had a headache. I couldn't get comfy enough to sleep for more than an hour at a time. I had chest pain and swollen legs and Arthur did move less at some times than others. It was back to reading the tea leaves. Arthur's life depended on my ability to interpret these bodily signs, to judge when to sound the alarm, when I'd never been pregnant before and was not medically trained and had no idea what the 'normal' level of feeling ill was supposed to be. I was afraid of making an unnecessary fuss and afraid of the hospital, precariously balancing those fears against the fact that, if I made the wrong call, Arthur could die.

'I have some good news,' Eric added, getting up. 'You've been discharged from social services.'

'What? I haven't seen social services.'

He hovered a moment, then sighed and lowered himself back into the chair.

'The referral that was done because of your bipolar. But they've checked things out and said they're happy not to keep you on their books, so that's got to be a weight off your mind.'

'I didn't know about any of this.'

'Oh, yes, you would have done. Your midwife would have told you when she did the referral. At your first appointment.'

'No. This is the first I've heard of it.'

Eric had started recording the conversation in my maternity notes in real time. His eyes were fixed on what he was writing, but I didn't need to see them to know that he didn't believe me. I thought referring to social services without telling me was a dick move. Stella wouldn't have done that. I was right not to trust that first midwife. Horrible woman. I didn't say any of this out loud in case Eric wrote it down.

Once he was out of sight, I exhaled sharply. My heart was banging again, and I realised I'd been holding my breath.

———

Arthur's nursery was ready and waiting. The cot that had originally housed Jon and his siblings was reassembled and painted pale green. A mobile hung above it. Arthur's name was spelled out in coloured bunting along one wall – Jon's sister had sewn that for him – and an old friend of mine from Maplewood had painted a rainbow and hot-air balloon across another. Boxes of nappies were stacked beside the changing table. Tiny babygros hung in the wardrobe. It was all there, everything except him.

At night I sat on the edge of the bed in our attic bedroom, looking up through the slanted roof window at the great and gleaming moon. Every night it was a little fuller, a little rounder. What did Arthur look like? I wondered.

Birth announcements started to trickle in from the

antenatal group, reports from a far-off country. Birth, like death, was the great unknown, and we crossed the threshold one by one. Hayley had a boy and did not name him William. She, too, was on the other side. The group started to congregate there, to re-form through emails sent in the middle of the night.

All this time, even since before I knew I was pregnant, I had been moving steadily towards a precipice. There was no slowing and no stopping. I could only prepare and hope for the best. I hoped that I could trust my body to know what to do. I still hoped we could ride it out at home, although I'd made careful arrangements to dash down the road at the first sign of trouble. I hoped that Stella could be there. She had booked her shifts based on our best guesses, and Lisa was waiting in the wings. I hoped for a good beginning. Somehow or other, Arthur would be with us soon.

three

Failure to Progress

The most merciful thing in the world, I think, is the inability of the human mind to correlate all its contents.
H. P. Lovecraft, 'The Call of Cthulhu'[1]

February 2014

I'm not sure what happened that week, although I have all the jigsaw pieces here in front of me in a stack of medical notes, jotted down at the time by midwives and doctors and the like. It's three inches thick. I've sorted the notes into chronological order, and I've been through them with two different midwives. I know that Arthur was born by emergency caesarean section, category one – *'immediate threat to the life of the woman or foetus'* – on Thursday at 12.05 p.m., or possibly 12.11 p.m. I know that the reason cited was my *'failure to progress'*.

There are the facts, and there are inconsistencies that melt the facts away.

There are moments I remember, and there are the great gaps between them.

I've spent so long trying to translate these medical notes

into a narrative, to thread on those little beads of memory. I can make the notes tell a story, but that doesn't make it my story. I don't have a story so much as I have snapshots. I'll show you my snapshots, and I'll show you the fraying threads between.

———

There's my due date, a Saturday. It's the day we moved back into our house, having been chased out by rising flood waters a few days before. We stayed in a friend's flat up the hill until the water stopped, four doors down the road, and started to slowly recede.

There we are, Jon and I, removing the bricks from underneath the sofa, the sandbags against the front door. There's us inflating the birth pool in the front room, me posing for a photo with it, enormous.

There's us eating a roast dinner at the kitchen table on Sunday evening, playing Scrabble afterwards. There's me crowing because I've just played MEERKAT on a triple word score. There's that strange gushing feeling and there I am, waddling off to the loo and then waddling back. 'It's show time.' I am nervous, and excited, and pleased with my disgusting pun. That's when it starts.

And there I am, tossing and turning all Sunday night, my body surging and aching.

There's me waving Jon off to work early Monday morning, yelling after him that he needs to keep his phone on loud *and* vibrate.

There's me bouncing on my inflatable ball, humming, waiting, breathing deeply into the surges as they come.

The day wears on, contractions still irregular but more and more painful. My lower back hurts. I'm so tired already.

I'm lying on the sofa, legs akimbo, gritting my teeth while Stella rummages around. I just need to know that there's some progress. A centimetre or two. If I know that, I can keep going.

There's no progress, none at all. Not only is my cervix not dilated, it's hardly begun to think about it. I am not in labour. It would be generous to call it pre-labour. This could go on for days.

I press on. I press on and on and on, through Monday alone and through Tuesday with Jon by my side. We've got the TENS machine out. It buzzes away on my back like a dozen dying houseflies and it helps a bit.

We're timing the contractions on an app. The pain is worse, like being split open over and over at three-minute intervals. Or are they four-minute intervals? Labour, like every joke, is all about timing. Two contractions in ten minutes means you're not getting anywhere, while three contractions in ten minutes means there's an end in sight. We move around the empty house, room to room, with the app and the TENS machine and its wires and the water I'm trying to remember to sip.

When we phone the hospital, they ask about the timing, but it hurts too much to keep time properly, and it hurts in between ... I'm told to take paracetamol and to have a bath. I'm not in labour: this is *the latent phase*. What the hell is labour going to be like?

Now it's night-time. The curtains are drawn, and the front room is lit by candles, all along the mantelpiece. I am in the empty birth pool. It isn't time to fill it yet, but the contractions come in waves like flood water, pain that wrecks and washes everything away. My body is thrown against the sides of the pool. My face smacks into the plastic, that rubbery smell, my mouth open in shock, drowning, over and over.

Outside in the street a woman is screaming, howling in pain and terror like a hunted animal. It occurs to me that someone should find out who is screaming in the street at night. Someone should go out to help her.

Then I realise I am the woman screaming.

The mind and body separate, smoothly slide apart.

The mind floats upward, hovers two inches below the ceiling.

The mind watches the body, thrashing and kicking.

The mind laughs a small laugh and says: 'You are on your own, mate.'

The mind simply snaps like a twig underfoot, so quietly that no one notices.

Jon is on the phone. He says, 'What? Sorry, I can't ... Yeah, yeah, that's her.'

He tells me the midwife is on her way.

When the midwives come, there are two of them, and one is Stella. I should be relieved that Stella is here, but I am not me and she is not her. Everyone is an actor playing themselves in a surreal piece of avant-garde theatre entitled No One Knows What's Happening Any More. I hear myself say that I will do anything for the pain to stop and can I have some pethidine please.

Pethidine is kept at the hospital, so in we go. I don't know how we get there or what happens when we do. I do know that I'm only one centimetre dilated, and therefore I'm not in labour. They are taking me in as a special favour, or as an act of mercy. Really, I should be able to manage this with a bath and some paracetamol.

Fuck paracetamol, I think, sleepily, becoming aware of

myself again. I'm in a hospital bed, sparse and strange and unbedlike, in an otherwise empty room. I have white sticky tape on my inner arm, with a long tube trailing from underneath, hooked up to an IV drip. On a trolley is a large plastic jug of water, and a little disposable cup. I take great gulps. The water is tepid but lovely.

The pethidine is lovely too. My back still hurts, but I don't mind. Someone fetches me another jug of water and tells me I must drink it down before I go home because my heart is beating too fast. I start to slowly pace the room, swaying and leaning into the contractions as they come. I spill water down my dress as the strength of one takes me by surprise. Things are gearing up again.

I am told to come back when I'm in labour. Four centimetres. Four times further along than I am now.

I am in the attic bedroom with Jon and Lisa. The room is a little island, a mezzanine between earth and sky. The moon watches at the slanted roof window but it's washed out by daylight, barely there.

I'm on all fours like a cow on the linoleum floor while Lisa stretches a wide scarf across my belly, pulling it from side to side. Something is wrong. I know it, Stella knew it, everyone seems to know it – but we don't know what or why. Lisa thinks that Arthur might be facing the wrong way round, in which case my body will need to turn him before he can be born. That's what the scarf is for. I try to keep still as waves of pain crash through me.

My bed is a cloud, and I am curled into it. Lisa massages my lower back hard, pressing her thumbs as if to pin me down, to keep me from being swept away.

'Don't stop,' I beg through gritted teeth. I have to trust her not to stop.

Now it's dark. I'm writhing in the back of Lisa's car, the seatbelt slicing into my neck as I thrash about. The engine growls. Every bump, every turn is agony. I'm done. Anything for this to be over. I don't care what happens so long as this is over.

Under hospital lights, I clutch a plastic mask to my face. Gas and air. I take one gasp, and vomit bile like battery acid across the room. Water cools my burning throat. I am trembling.

I've had more pethidine, and pain unclenches its great jaw, no longer chewing me up. I sip water as negotiations are under way in the delivery room. The midwives want a urine sample so that they can do a dip-stick test, but I can't wee. They want to know when I last had a wee and I have no idea. I am sent to the toilet 'for a try' like a toddler between sips of water.

Lisa is trying to feed me hot cross buns. I'm so thankful, not because I want a hot cross bun – in fact, this is probably the first time in my life I've refused a hot cross bun – but because Jon is visibly exhausted, and Lisa is a little candle in this vast and nightmarish landscape.

I finally have that wee. 'Did you manage it?' calls a midwife from behind the door.

'Um, yeah … it's mostly blood. I assume that's not good?'

It is, indeed, not good. There is talk of urine infections and kidney infections and antibiotics and the need for a blood test.

Time has jumped again. It moves in little leaps like a startled rabbit. For a while people have been sticking needles into me without success, but I've hardly noticed. I'm assured that it's all right because the senior anaesthetist has been called and he'll be able to get some blood, no problem.

The senior anaesthetist rolls up like a rock star: a bald man in scrubs exuding confidence, a definite swagger in his gait.

'Settle down, everybody. Papa's here.'

He doesn't quite say that but it's close.

I take one look at him, framed in the doorway with his hands on his hips, and half shout, 'What fresh hell is this!' I feel drunk, strangely exhilarated. I swear pethidine wasn't like this last time. What a bonus. Everyone pretends they haven't heard me, but Jon stifles a laugh, which makes me laugh too. It's a circus. Whose circus? I wonder. And whose monkeys?

I'm reclining on an examination table like an Ancient Roman at a banquet. The senior anaesthetist flashes me a grin as he sits down.

'Right,' he says. 'Let's get this done.'

Forty-five minutes later his head is gleaming with perspiration. He is a torch under the fierce lights, muttering expletives under his breath. He pretends I haven't heard him quite audibly call one of the veins in the back of my hand a motherfucker. It's monstrously funny. It's even funnier because I keep interrupting him to lurch my body forwards as a contraction takes me away for a few moments, hurtles me towards a distant shore.

I am the human pincushion. I could put spikes in all those punctures and be a porcupine.

I don't have any blood. I must have pissed out the last of it earlier. I'm a tangle of dry tunnels looping around and around. Dust blows through me. Desert winds. They're so loud I can't believe no one else can hear them.

Jon is staring at the wall. I can see he wants to be sick. I start to reassure him, but it strikes me how funny that is, given the circumstances, and I'm not sure if I've made sense.

The senior anaesthetist leaves the room, fists clenched. He is almost sulking. He says he will be back shortly.

Now they're looking at my cervix again. I should charge admission. I'd be like Scrooge McDuck.

'Congratulations,' drifts a voice from between my legs. I briefly wonder if I've had a baby and didn't notice, but no – it's that I am four centimetres dilated. 'You're in labour!'

This is funnier than anything that's happened yet. Let the games begin.

The midwife asks if I want an epidural. I consider it. Either the pethidine is wearing off or the news has sobered me up, but I'm back to myself for a moment.

I say, 'Give me four hours. If there's progress, then maybe I can do this.'

I really want to do this.

For four hours we do everything we can. I kneel at the end of the examination table and focus, riding waves of stinging, searing brine. I'm picturing revolving babies and my body opening and Arthur's scan photos, and I cry quiet tears as Jon paces the room and Lisa soothes and encourages and massages my lower back. The pain is worse and worse. I am seasick, retching but empty. I still don't want a hot cross bun.

The next viewing of my cervix feels momentous. The room is crowded suddenly. Everyone has gathered on the shore, waiting for news. I stare into the ceiling tiles, and I breathe deeply, my toes curled tight.

'Still four centimetres, I'm afraid.'

'Is there any progress?' I hear that I am pleading. 'Anything at all?'

'No, not really. I'm sorry.'

It's been four days and I am done. I'm so far beyond my limit and it's obvious to everyone that I am going to have to call it. I call it. They take me away.

From there, the memories are fewer and further between, fevered snatches of a bad dream.

I'm trying to keep still for the epidural and not thrash about, but I'm being wrung like a flannel. They cannot thread the catheter.

'*Pain ++*,' someone has written. '*Decision to resite.*'

I sleep a little. The world fractures into smaller and smaller pieces, these smashed-up smithereens of time.

Lisa sits alone, dozing in the half-light. She smiles at me across the room and says that Jon has gone to find some coffee.

There's a clip attached to Arthur's head, monitoring his heart rate, and it keeps coming off. They reattach it over and over. Hot, white slices of pain darting up and into me. Stuffing me with shards of glass. Screams jam in my throat. I thought the epidural meant the pain would stop.

'Must be a duff bag of clips,' someone mutters in the darkness.

I am still not dilating. They increase the dose of Syntocinon to make the contractions stronger and more frequent, then increase it again. They record five contractions every ten minutes.

I am so thirsty. My tongue is thick, fuzzy felt. My eyes sting. I blink hard to focus my vision. I can't move. There's no context, no meaning, no moment before or after this one. There's only the thirst.

Faces hover over me, bobbing in and out of view. I'm trying to speak, to ask for water, but my tongue is stuck fast. My lips part uselessly. I plead with my eyes, but no one notices. They're busy with something. They're speaking a language I don't understand.

I recognise Jon. His face and voice are suddenly so clear. 'I think she's thirsty.'

Jon stands over me with a white disposable cup and, in that moment, he is Jesus Christ, Buddha, and all four of the Beatles rolled into one. My head is heavy, but I manage to lift it a little, and Jon holds the cup to my lips. I would weep with relief if my eyes weren't so sticky. I anticipate cool water, any second now . . .

It spills, soaking into my hospital gown. I didn't get to taste it. I wish that I could die.

Jon is back, with a bright-pink plastic straw in another cup of water.

I manage the smallest sip before the next contraction comes and everything rolls away on a tide of unknowing.

I am eight centimetres dilated and being told to stop pushing. I'm not pushing. My body is pushing.

I am ten centimetres dilated and my body is still pushing but now I'm trying to join in. A midwife records that she is '*coaching*' me and that I am '*pushing well*'.

I push for four more hours. The word *push* fills my being. *Push. Push. Push.* I don't know what I'm pushing, or why, or what this is all for. I'm a body in a bed. Someone notes that my heart rate has reached 200 bpm.

The room fills with scrubs and white coats and whispers in corners. A woman waves a piece of paper in my face. She tells me that I need to sign it and I blink at her, uncomprehending.

'Your name,' she urges. 'We need you to write your name.'
I try to work out what she means. My name . . .

—

I don't remember much after that. I was wheeled into theatre. Jon changed into scrubs and followed, but I don't recall his being there. Lisa was left behind. She phoned my mum in tears. The doctors attempted a forceps delivery, tearing me in the process and injuring Arthur's face. They didn't realise that the epidural hadn't worked properly, that I felt it all. Thank god they numbed me with a spinal block before cutting me open.

I knew that something important was happening. I needed to stay awake, to be present, but as pain evaporated from my body, the tide was pulling me away more relentlessly than before. I struggled against it, kicking to stay afloat, but my legs didn't move. Water swept over my face. I drifted in and out as Arthur was born. They wrapped him and placed him on my chest, but my head was so heavy I couldn't lift it to see him.

Arthur floated away from me amid voices, the whirring of a vacuum, a wind that whipped around the room. I fell backwards and sank gratefully into the dark sea.

The Mother-Creature

*Here I am, in borrowed bones, in makeshift skin, looking out
of eyes that are a construct, breathing with lungs that are only
a step – a basic arrangement – away from leaves. How funny,
to have a body when I am not a body? How funny to be inside
when I am outside?*

Helena Fox, *How It Feels to Float*[1]

February to March 2014

My body washed up, pale and swollen, on a bed in
the postnatal ward.

Miraculously, the bloated thing began to move and
speak. Leaking, incontinent, weeping at nothing, it could
neither walk nor stand, but it rapidly learned to mimic me.
It made phone calls. It held whole conversations. It made
sure to say that it – that I – was so in love, and that Arthur
was beautiful.

I suppose he was beautiful, if rather battered-looking.
Someone had put him in a cot that was a transparent plastic box on wheels beside the bed. He lay there, quite
unconscious, flat on his back with froggy arms and legs

bent at right angles by his side. Berry-coloured scabs and bruises were forming on his head, and across one side of his face was a dark claw mark. His expression was oblivion. He coughed and made little mucusy noises from time to time, but he slept and didn't wake.

This corpse, this mother-body, wept and fussed and stared straight through him.

Meanwhile I was fathoms deep, curled close and tight in the darkness.

They wrote, '*Laura feeling generally well, though exhausted.*' Someone had sketched a drawing of where the incision across my pelvis had ripped as Arthur was hauled into the world, and where that tear was in relation to my bladder. Blood loss was estimated at 1.5 litres.

When a new scribe took over, they began by citing my '*failure to progress*'. This was the justification for a caesarean section, or the reason it had come to that. The phrase is on almost every page. Everything that happened had its origins there, in the fact that I had failed at this most basic, most essential task.

The mother-creature, who was me and not me, drifted in and out on the tide.

That evening, Jon was sent home. I was responsible for feeding the baby and changing his nappy every three hours overnight. That was when it became apparent that I was losing time. I would look at the clock above the door, turn towards the window, look back, and it might be five seconds later, or twenty minutes, or an hour, or four. Had I fallen asleep? I couldn't hold on to threads of thought long enough to wonder.

In odd moments, I realised that the baby sleeping beside me needed to be fed, but I was trapped, immobile. I pressed the buzzer for help and a midwife stuck her head around the door on her way past.

'I'll be right back,' she called.

And time had moved again. Press buzzer and repeat. Press buzzer and repeat.

At 9 a.m. Arthur was fed and changed by a midwife who noted that he was dehydrated and wrote, '*Encouraged Laura to call for assistance when needed.*'

After a day or two, they moved us off the postnatal ward and into a side room. Normally you would have to pay for the luxury of privacy and extra space, but the room was empty and, as we wouldn't be going home for a while, they gave it to us. I think it was an act of kindness.

Our new family of three hovered in limbo between birth and home. Soon there was a steady stream of visitors: Arthur's grandparents and godparents and uncles and aunts. They brought gifts – we had such an abundance of gifts – and took photos of each other holding the baby. No one seemed to realise that I wasn't there. Arthur slept on and on.

My mother-double took her first shuffling steps. She became more adept, more convincing. She needed to be. Arthur had a tongue-tie, which is when the frenulum – the little strip of skin connecting the tongue to the bottom of the mouth – is too short and so movement of the tongue is restricted. The first we heard of it was when a doctor came with a red book, a health record for keeping track of immunisations and weigh-ins.

'When a tongue-tie is only slight,' she said, handing over the red book, 'we tend to leave them and see how it goes, but this is a major one. It'll have to be snipped.'

'Snipped?'

'Yes. They'll snip it with a pair of scissors.'

You can get away from my baby with your scissors, I might have thought, or said. The creature in my place just nodded.

Every three hours, she roused Arthur and poked a bottle of formula into his mouth. It took an hour or more to get 20 mls into his baby-bird gape. His face puckered with effort, as if sucking thick milkshake through a thin straw, and he promptly fell back asleep. The midwives taught her to tickle his feet, tickle his chin, every trick in the book, but Arthur seemed as reluctant to be there as I was.

The mother-creature rose to the task. She was made for this, born out of death to weep and worry, love and feed. Still, she dreaded the close of every three-hour interval, dreaded trying to keep him alert, to coax him to try, while the minutes crawled by and the milk level in the bottle went down in minuscule amounts. She asked again about the tongue-tie snip, and was told that, because she wasn't breastfeeding, Arthur was 'not a priority'. Once discharged home, she was to ask the GP for a referral. The waiting list was around nine months.

The creature wept in her little room, quite apart from a world she had never belonged to or even encountered. She, too, fell asleep unexpectedly. When visitors came to admire the baby, Jon often had to take them elsewhere. Hours were misplaced like squares of white muslin, lost because they were all alike.

Arthur's face became peakier and sallower until he was noticeably orange: jaundice, because he was underfed. The treatment was phototherapy. A metal machine with a halogen lamp, not unlike an overhead projector, was wheeled in. Arthur was stripped to his nappy and placed under its glare. He had a little mask to protect his eyes, but he would wriggle, still asleep, and the mask would shift, so he needed someone to sit and watch and keep putting the mask back in place.

At around 10 p.m., the door swished open. A midwife entered briskly with her clipboard and surveyed the scene – the mother-creature dozing, the baby under the lamp, Jon on mask duty, keeping watch. Like a schoolteacher who has caught a rule-breaker in the act, she told Jon in her emphatic Canadian accent that it wasn't visiting hours and he was to leave immediately. Jon made his case: we were in a private room and not disturbing anyone; I'd had a bad time and needed to rest; Arthur was under the lamp and needed watching because of the mask . . . The midwife listened in silence, lips pursed, and then asked if she should call security and have Jon 'forcibly removed'. He went out, fuming, into the night.

The mother-creature hauled herself off the bed and she sat beside that lamp all night long, digging her fingernails into her palms to stay awake. The nails left crescent moons, red like the first light of dawn as it blurred the edges of the window blinds. The sky was raging, sore and inflamed, that morning, but the blinds held against it. There were only smudges of light on the walls, arranged around the halogen lamp and the glowing, starving child beneath.

The midwife returned, holding the door open with one foot and leaning in to issue instructions. The baby was to go back in his cot and the phototherapy unit to be wheeled out into the corridor. She was already closing the door when the mother-creature piped up faintly. The machine was plugged into the floor, and she couldn't bend to unplug it, and it was heavy . . . Her voice, faltering, trailed off.

'It's important to keep active after a caesarean,' the midwife said curtly, and left.

The mother-creature could have gone back to bed. Really, she should have gone back to bed. No one could have actually forced her to bend to the plug socket, or to start lugging machinery about. There were many good reasons not to attempt it. I like to think that if I had been there, if I had been myself, I would have told the midwife to get fucked. At the same time, it was me in that room – it can hardly have been anyone else – and I did as I was told. It took a few hours.

I think my friend Julie was the first to sense how broken I was, almost literally fractured in two – or at least that something was quite seriously 'off' – when she came to visit us the following day. Julie and I had met at the pub and become close over late-night pints. She said, later, that she was hesitant to draw conclusions, as she wasn't sure what people were usually like soon after they have babies, but that I looked absent. I talked about all the awful things that had happened and were still happening as one talks about the weather.

I don't remember that, but I do remember we were mid-conversation when a midwife came in with a clipboard and said that she needed to ask me about contraception.

'Ooh, shall I—' Julie started, picking up her bag and making as if to scuttle out of the room, but I waved away the need for this. Never had sex been less on the cards, even hypothetical future sex. My catheter had just been taken out. Typically, I might have said something like, 'I think I'm going to be favouring the Get-The-Fuck-Away-From-Me method for quite some time . . .'

But I wasn't there, not really. Although the bloated doppelgänger in the bed had my voice and face, and although by this time she could do most of what I could do, she would never quite master honesty. She mumbled something vague about condoms. The midwife dutifully wrote this down. Everyone smiled and hoped that the midwife would leave, and she did.

As the door clicked shut behind her, Julie said, 'Wow. I wouldn't have dared ask you that, not right now,' and she looked at me with an odd expression on her face.

For a moment, I stirred on an ocean-bed, tasting salt and seeing the silhouetted outline of my hair trailing above me in the dark.

Another moment and I was in my body, in that bed, in the maternity wing of that hospital, in that town, right at the centre of a succession of things-within-things, a Russian doll.

I looked around at Julie and Jon, and then at the baby fast asleep. That baby was my baby. My Arthur. It seemed inconceivable.

I looked down at my wax hands, fat fingers like raw sausages, the great swollen bulk of my lap.

Then I closed my eyes, and I was gone.

———

That evening, Stella came in. 'Oh, Laura,' she said when she saw me. There was a pause. 'Look, I'm on tonight. Shall I have Arthur with me in the office? Keep it quiet – we're not supposed to do it any more – but you look like you need the sleep.'

I did sleep, and the next day we were all a bit brighter – or, in Arthur's case, less bright and more flesh-coloured. There were murmurs of discharging us home. This was all very well, but the tongue-tie clearly needed snipping sooner rather than later, and no one was allowed to do it because there was a separate 'clinical pathway' for bottle-fed babies.

It was as if I were being punished for not breastfeeding. Worse, it was as if Arthur were being punished. It didn't matter that I was following medical advice so that I could continue to take medication. It didn't matter that I'd lost a lot of blood and was anaemic. It didn't matter that, because of everything that had happened, it was unlikely that breastfeeding would have been a success even if I'd tried. It didn't even seem to matter that Arthur, who had no say in the matter whatsoever, was ill because he wasn't getting the milk that his little body so desperately needed.

After some discussion, a baby-feeding specialist arrived to watch me give Arthur his bottle. He had perked up since going under the lamp and would feed for a few minutes at a time. As he drank, he made a harsh ticking noise, milk dribbling down his chin. I couldn't keep dabbing at it while also holding him and the bottle, so the muslin I'd tucked into his babygro was drenched. The specialist brought another specialist, who wrote: '*Slurping noise and clucking noise* ↑ *loud.*'

Everyone agreed that the procedure should be done urgently but their hands, like Arthur's tongue, were tied. The only leverage we had, the only justification considered, was that a tongue-tie division would enable us to go home. It would, in their words, 'clear the bed'.

The mother-creature sat tight in the unclear bed, scouring the internet on her phone. She went on the tongue-tie practitioners' website and phoned every private tongue-tie practitioner in the country. No one could help any time soon. She phoned breastfeeding groups and lactation specialists who did tongue-tie snips. Arthur would not be welcome. The mother-creature was polite. She understood. She only became more lifelike, more entrenched where she was.

I was still somewhere, twitching from time to time, groping, treading water. But I had been forgotten. I was the mother-creature now.

The bed was cleared when someone at the hospital 'pulled some strings', and we were discharged home with a tongue-tie appointment for the following day.

As I stepped outside for the first time in over a week, daffodils crowded the grassy mounds around the hospital buildings once again. Arthur had brought the spring with him. He looked impossibly small, strapped into his car seat, where he slept scrunched up like a hedgehog. Jon pored over the car-seat instruction manual. I carried the gift bags, stuffed with antibiotics and iron tablets and codeine, nestled among bright tissue paper.

When I returned to our attic bedroom, it smelt sour, and I found that someone – or something – had bitten a hole in the duvet.

Arthur's tongue-tie was snipped on the neonatal unit, among babies in incubators, babies you could have held in one hand, in an atmosphere of dread hush. It took seconds. He cried only for a moment, settling straight back to sleep in my arms. Then we left and never went back.

A week passed, days leaking and staining and blending into one another like watercolours. More visitors. We were so fortunate to have this large, supportive network of friends and family. Our freezer was full of cooked meals. There were more presents and offers to babysit. And yet everyone was a stranger because I was someone else, someone who hadn't existed until recently. I could only smile and say thank you.

Stella came most days. I don't know how she managed it, with the restrictions around her and demands on her time, but she kept coming over, kept writing down the same things: '*Laura appears pale and tired.*'

I felt pale, insubstantial, as if I might drift through walls or fall through the floor. There were times when the world went skittering away, bouncing like a stone thrown over water. It was fitting, somehow, this ghostly existence. I had met death and come halfway back. I could only ever be half present, exhausted by making myself manifest.

Then, one day, I left Arthur with Jon, took to my bed, and stayed there. I was so cold, brittle with cold, my thigh-bones rods of ice under the covers. My skin crumbled to powder when the light touched it. I dreamed hundreds of years had passed and I was hauled out of the earth, miraculously preserved.

I staggered to the toilet and, in a moment of inspiration, rummaged for paracetamol and a thermometer. As I half fell back into bed, the thermometer was still wedged under my tongue, beeping insistently. I texted Stella: '*Thermometer says 39.1. Is that okay?*' and sank into a fitful doze.

The next I remember I was in hospital again, being inter-
rogated about vaginal discharge. Was it yellow? Brown?
Foul-smelling? I had no idea. This body and I really were not
that intimate. Someone wrote that my scar was healing well,
but my abdomen was tender and hot. I hadn't noticed. I
sounded so stupid, trying to answer their questions. I could
have said, 'Look, I don't live here any more,' but I didn't
know, just as dead people don't know that they're dead. My
whole experience of everything – of being myself, in a body,
in time – had shifted, but I couldn't remember any different.
This was just how it was.

When the memory of what happened next first came
to me, I dismissed it as a fever dream, but the trusty stack
of medical notes bears witness. Dr James arrived, the first
time I'd seen her since early in my pregnancy.

'I heard all about the birth,' she said. 'We were worried
there, for a bit. You know, I've never lost a patient.'

I've never lost a me, either. My former self might have
mentioned this, but the mother-creature just smiled.

Dr James repeated all the questions I'd already been
asked and failed to satisfactorily answer, then proceeded to
explain why she was asking. I had an infection, she said,
but it wasn't clear whether the infection was external, in
my caesarean wound, or internal, in my uterus. 'Lie back,
and I'll have a good look.'

She walked slowly, pulling the curtain around us in our
strange intimacy. I felt the crisp bedsheets brush against
my skin. The ceiling tiles were whitish-grey, pockmarked,
the light glaring and blurring.

In her hand, Dr James held what looked like a crochet
hook.

Pain looped through me, from my belly and out into

my fingers and toes, into my tongue, trailing telephone wire, sharp as splintered bone. The bed dropped beneath me, and then all feeling drained away. It left a sensation of floating, as if I were levitating. I didn't make a sound, and I lay quite still as Dr James unravelled me, her hook picking and poking and rummaging, threads trailing down the bed, onto the floor, across the ward, out into the corridor. I went with them, letting the dark tide of forgetting take me all over again.

If I saw an apparition, it wasn't an angel or spirit. What came to me in that moment were Rose and Florence, two teddy bears Nan knitted for me when I was small. I was into Florence Nightingale at the time, and I'd requested that Florence be a nurse. Nan had kitted her out in a blue dress and white pinafore, but she was less of a success than Rose, being rather angular. She looked not so much like a nurse as a hammerhead shark. Both teddies were stuffed with Nan's old tights and, if you squinted, you could just about see tights through the dozens of tiny holes.

I saw Nan's hands, mottled with age but moving at miraculous speed, needles clicking. I gave her my own mangled knitting and she unpicked it, the long strand of wool dropping down to the carpet.

How strange it is that a human being can be stitched, and unpicked, and restitched – or not – at will.

'Sorry, this must hurt,' Dr James offered, grimly. 'Let me just—' I heard her suck in air through her teeth, and yet she was so far away.

'I'm fine,' I heard myself say. 'Don't worry.'

I was to have antibiotics on a drip for a few days. They kept me on the postnatal ward, and I could have had

Arthur with me, but I chose to leave him at home with Jon. The mother-creature was losing her grip.

—

I came home with more tablets and little pots of luminous medicine. Some had to be kept in the fridge, but I could never remember which, nor could I keep track of when to take what. Some antibiotics were for five days, some for seven, but the days of the week were so slippery and would not keep their place in the queue. I relied on a complicated series of alarms on my phone, getting up at night to take medicine as well as to see to Arthur.

In the dim light, in the small hours, my mother-double and I were crammed together in this body, neither dead nor alive. She was a dumb, lovesick, compliant sort of creature, and even she began to be torn from me, wrenched back into oblivion. Everything was slowly sliding into an abyss. Lost hours became lost days, and I was becoming simply no one. The cruellest thing about it wasn't even that I continued walking around, talking, mothering, and that nobody knew. It was that I didn't know.

I kept a baby journal and mechanically wrote words of love I couldn't feel or even comprehend. I like to think that some part of me, somewhere, meant them, but when I look back, it's as if I wasn't there. I have photos, but I don't recognise Arthur or myself. I had never felt the 'rush of love' that my mum described, but then I don't think I felt anything much, nor had I noticed the absence. How much I could recall of the previous few weeks seemed to vary from hour to hour, but most of what I've described in these chapters didn't emerge until later. This amnesia may have been a mercy, but it was going to cause problems.

When the Bough Breaks

I walked home, heartsore, through pale streets,
the coins of Motherhood singing in my pockets.
    Liz Berry, 'The Republic of Motherhood'[1]

March to April 2014

Perhaps we shut off from our bodies when we know that they're dying. Perhaps that's the first stage of death. If that's true, I think it works in reverse as well. If we're lucky enough that our bodies begin to mend themselves, sooner or later they'll show up to reclaim us.

Jon had used up his paternity leave and all available annual leave, so he had to go back to work, but I wasn't up to caring for Arthur alone. I hadn't yet walked beyond the house. Thankfully my mum was able to take compassionate leave from her job as a teaching assistant, and she came up from Southampton to stay with us. She cleaned the kitchen and helped me push the pram to Sainsbury's down the road. We took our time over coffee there, so that I could have a rest before heading home.

Every day I was a little more mobile. People started telling me I looked better. There was an appointment with Dr Freyman, who wrote to the GP that he had no concerns for my mental health. The time came for Stella to discharge us from midwifery care. On her final visit, she said, 'I knew you wouldn't get postnatal depression.'

This was all very promising, except for the fact that I was still sleepwalking.

As my body recovered, as Stella stopped coming, as Mum went home, I began to revisit myself, briefly, to dip a toe in the water. At first it wasn't so bad. At first it only happened at night. Arthur's cry would rouse me, piercing the darkness until the whole attic room seemed bright, ringing with his need. I'd lift him from the Moses basket beside the bed and bring him down to the nursery, so that Jon could sleep, and I'd feed him his bottle in the rocking chair beside the window. It was just us, then. The moon hung like a lamp behind the curtain, growing dim and sleepy as he fed. I gazed into Arthur's calm, knowing little face, and that was when I heard my body calling me home.

It was distant at first, but as it came closer it was a rumble, then a roar. A sick, panicked, choking feeling. That was when I realised that something was wrong.

There were jarring moments when I would be back, suddenly, as myself. I caught glimpses of a woman, sleep-starved and desperate, who had to roll on her side to get out of bed, searing pain in her stitches, white baby-sick on her nightie, trapped. I ran as fast and as far as I could into nothingness, anything to get away from her. But the original version of me kept trying to stagger ashore, so that my two selves met face to face, a mirror image where the sea touched the land.

Time started to jump backwards as well as forwards.

I don't know if you, reading this, have ever had a flashback: it's like being in a time machine, but one that's controlled by someone else. There you are, washing up at the kitchen sink. The kettle is boiling, steam rises, and as it finishes there's a clean, clear *click* – and it's the sound of retching in the delivery room, as your stomach slaps wetly against the back of your throat. Your hair is clinging to your face with sweat. The lights are hot and humming. Greenish-yellow vomit drips down the wall. The plastic mask is hissing in the midwife's hand . . . And then you're back in your kitchen. You stand stupidly, up to your elbows in warm water for what seems like hours.

My imagination, which had always been my solace, became my tormentor. They're known as 'intrusive thoughts', those ideas and scenarios that rise unbidden and follow us around, like gum stuck to a shoe. It's not uncommon, or so I'm told. People stand on the edge of a train-station platform and think, I could jump. They see a pigeon on the pavement and think, I could kick that pigeon. Or not. Maybe that one's just me. Sometimes I picture myself shouting something embarrassing on the bus or responding to kindness with a bizarre rude entitlement. I'm assured that many of us have thoughts like that. These images flit in and out and they curl our toes, but we live with them.

At least, I lived with them until the theatre between my ears ran a season of vignettes themed around the idea of me – or some shadowy, anonymous figure that *might be me* – doing the most creatively cruel things to baby Arthur. I'd like to describe these to you, offer an example, but I find that even now I can't voice them. Even my typing fingers do not want to go there. They were – are – so graphic and distressing. The possibility that they might be premonitions, or that through sheer power of suggestion I might be seized by the impulse to act them out, left me abjectly terrified. I couldn't live with that.

Most of the time, I maintained outward composure. I may have been losing my mind, but I wasn't staggering around like Lear, far from it. As everything became wilder and more disintegrated internally, externally it was almost the opposite. Perhaps this was an unconscious survival strategy. Perhaps it was that there was a familiarity to it all. For me, the dance between what is and what has been and what might be has always been a lively one. A vivid memory and a technicolour imagination are gifts as much as they are burdens, but after Arthur was born, they ramped up to a point that was intolerable, that lent a sense of utter desperation to everything I did. It was a miracle no one seemed able to tell.

At first, I put it down to lack of sleep. There was still an issue with Arthur's tongue-tie. He was gaining weight, but clacking away loudly as he drank his bottle, and I spent hours winding him – long days and longer nights, holding him upright, walking around, rubbing his back, patting him, bouncing up and down. We bought these bottles and those bottles, these teats and those teats, colic drops, gripe water ... Anything that was going at the chemist, we tried it. Even when Arthur was asleep, having him beside us was like bedding down in a farmyard. He shifted and grunted and squeaked, a tiny, basketed gremlin. I was sure I would feel so much saner if I could only get some proper sleep.

I remember pacing around the kitchen with my phone to my ear, pleading with a GP who had just prescribed yet more medication for oral thrush. Arthur grizzled in his bouncy chair. His tongue was coated white, as if it had been snowing in his mouth. Jon had taken him to the GP appointment because I couldn't face it. He had asked about the tongue-tie, and the doctor was resolute that it wasn't an issue. When I phoned, the same doctor grudgingly conceded that if we were still having problems in a few weeks, we could come back to the surgery, and he'd consider making a referral so that Arthur could join the waiting list for the tongue-tie clinic. I told myself – and the doctor – incessantly that I just couldn't go on without sleep. That was true enough, but I think I also meant that I couldn't go on full stop.

It was Lisa who put me in touch with a breastfeeding support service called Nature's Mothers.* I was not one of nature's mothers, not entitled to that care, but I was going to take it anyway, for Arthur, if I could get it. I spoke on the phone to someone named Sarah, and we were invited to come to a drop-in session the following Thursday.

When Thursday came, the pram rattled over cobbled streets as I tried to steer it and navigate on my phone at the same time. We arrived at another red-brick building like a church hall, but this one was grander than where the antenatal classes were held, two storeys high. I parked my pram under the stairs and carried Arthur up with the changing bag slung over my shoulder, bulging suspiciously. I had packed it with bottles and teats and beakers of made-up formula. It felt illicit, like smuggling sweets into the cinema.

We came to a large, echoing room, where mothers and babies were gathered at one end. I took a seat with Arthur

---

* Nature's Mothers has since been renamed Lotus Midwife.

in my arms. It never occurred to me how funny it was, bashfully concealing the bottle beneath my cardigan as I sat among all these women with their breasts out. They had mugs of tea, some in a spare hand and some on the floor just out of reach, muslins and baby slings draped over their shoulders, biscuits balanced precariously on knees as they fed.

Was I also allowed tea and a biscuit? I wondered. I wasn't sure, because any tea and biscuits consumed would be just for me: I wouldn't be transmuting them into miracle milk for my baby. How selfish it must seem, I thought, and how strange to have refused the opportunity to offer my own child what was universally agreed to be the best nutrition. It was like I stank of it, the failure, first to birth Arthur and then to feed him as well. The source of his suffering located squarely at the fact that I had failed, was still failing, as his mum.

The shame I brought to the group was all my own. I was conspicuous, but never condemned. I had my tea and biscuit. Mothers sat around in twos or threes, or alone. I sat alone. Like little islands, we fed our babies, and rocked and shushed, while Sarah and her colleague moved quietly between us. Sarah was dark-haired, with an air of energy and capability about her. When she came to me, I wanted to hand Arthur over, to say, 'Here, take this. Clearly you can do this, but I can't. I'm not good enough for him.' Instead, I fear I might have vomited all sorts of details about the most harrowing events of the previous five weeks. At least, I remember a long conversation.

Sarah watched as I gave Arthur a bottle, then slipped her finger under his tongue. She said that the tongue-tie had re-emerged, and that this isn't unusual when they're snipped in the first ten days. She explained everything gently and thoroughly and asked me if I would like to go ahead with the procedure. I said yes please, and, again, it was very quick. It cost about a hundred quid, and I was conscious that I was fortunate to have a hundred quid going spare. I expect they would have helped us even if I didn't, and I hope my hundred quid helped to fund the same for someone else.

Two days after the tongue-tie snip, I started to bleed. What I had assumed to be my first post-baby period quickly became unmanageable. I swapped my menstrual pads for some maternity ones I found zipped into a pocket of my hospital bag. The next morning, I was soaking one every hour. By lunchtime, there were blood clots like squashed blackberries. I don't remember much after that, and so I turn, once again, to my stack of medical notes. If I could scrunch up all this photocopied paper and stuff it into the gaps, would it plug the holes in my story?

We went to A & E. A doctor had a look up there – and by 'up there' I refer, once again, to my vagina, which made more public appearances over those few months than ever before or since. In the notes, the doctor has written: '*Imp: Period. Plan: Home.*' I remember telling him that I'd never had a period like this before, and he said that the first period after birth is often heavier, and that it was probably heavier still because I wasn't breastfeeding. He recorded this fact alongside my temperature and blood pressure and underlined it for good measure.

I didn't query it again, even to myself. Just what you get, I thought, if you fuck up giving birth and don't even feed your own baby. Arthur had suffered; it seemed only right that I should suffer too.

I bled for the next three weeks. It *was* heavy: it weighed me down, tethered me. I planned my movements around the location of the nearest toilet, and I dreaded going because there was always so much blood. It soaked into everything. The bedsheets were ruined, all my underwear. I felt dizzy again, like a sketch of a person outlined in pencil.

Several years later, when I went through my birth and postnatal notes with a midwife, she said that this crime scene of a period was probably a secondary haemorrhage.

Somehow, I stayed on the move, my changing bag stuffed with maternity pads so I could swap them in supermarket toilets. I paced up and down the local high street with my pram, aimlessly, mindlessly, past all the shops, along the river and round ... The rhythmic plodding soothed Arthur and lulled me into an altered state, better to tune out the exhaustion, the cramping and dizziness, and my very great misery. Walking was an empty landscape, a sort of sleep. It took me away from the clenched fist of my body, grasping and squeezing, its habit of suckerpunching me into places I didn't want to be.

These sagas – the tongue-tie, bleeding, deterioration of my mental state, god knows what else – were playing out at the same time, but it was as if the parts of me who dealt with them were quite separate. They were strangers in different worlds, who lived and suffered in parallel with one another. There were still times when I simply wasn't there. There were other times when I had real insight into my situation, and then I was quite seriously concerned and at a loss to know what to do. I knew I was supposed to be vigilant for signs of postnatal depression, but I was also a seasoned enough madness veteran to know that I wasn't depressed. I knew how depression felt, and whatever was up with me felt different.

I asked for advice from other mums on Facebook. I felt uneasy about joining the postnatal ranks at mother and baby groups in libraries and children's centres, because I didn't feel like one of them. There had been no birth. There had been an operation. A bad dream. It wasn't the crossing of a threshold that I'd expected and that I assumed everyone else had just done. It was easier to be a new mum in that disembodied space with the women in my phone. They formed an invisible web that caught me as I fell.

It wasn't a psychiatrist, or a midwife, or a health visitor, but a single mother of three on a remote Scottish island who explained that birth trauma – postnatal post-traumatic stress – is a thing. To me, it was an alien concept. PTSD was for war veterans. People who survived natural disasters or violent assault might get a look-in, but having a baby is an ordinary event. Of course, this young mum I'd never met was bang on the money, and she did what none of the health professionals had known to do. She gave me an understanding of what I was facing.

She also said that I should talk to Jon about how I was feeling. Jon was working long hours, and even in bed beside me, he was so distant he may as well have been on the moon. He was doing his best. We both were. We were gritting our teeth and getting through it, separately. When we eventually came out the other side, we were both changed, and there was no getting back to one another.

What none of us knew – not me, not Jon, not our

well-established support network of local friends or my brand-new support network of virtual friends – was that I was in danger, and things were about to get much worse.

———

I don't know how they started, or where they came from, those sudden impulses to kill myself. What began as an intrusive thought became an idle daydream, the reassurance of an emergency exit. It created a strange sense of safety, knowing that I need not tolerate the intolerable, but this evolved all too quickly into a stony determination that I was going to end my life. The rationale was clear and compelling. I had to protect Arthur from any harm I might do to him in a moment of frenzy. I was no good for him, no good as a mother. And I was half dead already.

I couldn't shake the sense that I was rotting and disintegrating from the inside out. If I could bear to touch that scar across my pelvis, if I could rip it open with my fingernails, it would reveal a festering cavity. The decay was toxic, contaminating everything I touched – and I touched Arthur more than anything or anyone else. My kisses on the softness of his cheek, my fingers pressing the poppers on his babygro were poison. People say that suicide is selfish, but at the time I believed the selfish thing was to continue to inflict myself on everyone, and on Arthur most of all. He deserved so much better than this. He deserved so much better than me.

I don't know that I had much of a plan. I did make plans, but then I lost time and lost the opportunity with it. I remember standing at the far end of an empty train-station platform, watching for the next train passing at full speed. Arthur was sleeping in his pram. I placed a full bottle beside him, and I turned the pram away so that he wouldn't be facing me when I jumped, even though his eyes were closed. Then the curtain falls on that memory, but I can't have leapt in front of a train. I must have just gone home.

Every moment was a roll of the dice. It might be lights on and nobody home. It might be flashbacks and intrusive thoughts firing all over the place. I might be coldly suicidal. I might even be fine. Sometimes I seemed to exist in multiple states at once, as if I were two or three people jostling for space in this one battered body. One of them knew that it was all up to her: she had to steer herself and Arthur to safety before it was too late.

I could have contacted Annette at the community mental health service. I was still on her books, but the thought of seeing her was enough to nudge me over the edge of any station platforms I might find myself on. Instead, I spoke to my health visitor, although I don't remember much about her or the conversation except that she advised me to make a GP appointment. Dr James drifted back to me, then, and the antenatal clinic at the hospital. That was what I was supposed to do: if I felt concerned about my mental health, I was to see a GP. I phoned the surgery on a Friday afternoon and made an urgent appointment for Monday.

As the weekend wore on, I felt uneasy that I might have overreacted. I seemed all right. We spent Sunday afternoon in the pub, ate a roast lunch and played board games with our friends. Arthur was an easy companion, smiling his adorable new smile, happy to be fussed and passed around and to have his nappy changed on a mat on the floor of the ladies' loo. But as dusk fell and it was time to go home, I couldn't bear to leave. I couldn't bear to be alone in that house with Jon and the baby, and to face the long night ahead.

'You go on with Arthur,' I said to Jon. 'I'll catch you up in a bit.'

A few hours later, I'd exhausted every excuse. All the regulars were leaving or had left, and it was evident that I needed to get back to my baby, my husband, my responsibilities. I said an elongated goodbye to the landlady, stepped out into the half-lit street, and began to walk. The chilly night air took my breath in little snatches. A familiar light-headedness lifted me off my feet, and as I floated towards home, I acknowledged to myself that I had nothing, nothing left to give.

I couldn't go home. I had to go home. I couldn't go home. I had to go home.

That thought pendulum was still swinging as I reached the front door. I meant to go in, but my feet kept walking – past Sainsbury's, over the bridge that crossed the Thames, into town, past the shopping centre, then snaking around and around the dark streets, going nowhere. A resignation settled over me. My phone buzzed in my pocket, and I ignored it. My maternity pad was soaking through, and I ignored that too. My hands were curled and empty in the sleeves of my coat.

If I walked for long enough, I would wind down like a clockwork toy, and then I could rest, and it wouldn't matter where I was. Or I'd eventually reach the shoreline and wade out, where the sea would pick me up under my arms and carry me away. Except, of course, that I didn't live near the sea any more, I had no idea where the sea was in relation to where I was, and my route looped round on itself endlessly, like circling a drain.

The river loomed in front of me and then I was halfway across the bridge, where I finally came to a stop. Below, streetlamps were reflected in the surface of the water like fireflies in a night sky. I stepped up to the railing and gripped the cold metal bars.

When I used to trespass on the top floor of the school manor house, the former asylum, I hauled myself up on the bars on the windows and looked out over the lumbering countryside. It was that same feeling of being tethered on an invisible rope – to the bridge, to the school, to the vast world. I felt light-headed and it was the lightness of girlhood, not having a pram, nor a plan, nor even a name. I might flutter on the breeze and sail upward like a discarded paper bag. What did any of it matter? I pictured the black water enveloping me, its cold finality closing over my head. And I thought, I'm going to jump off this bridge, because what else can I do?

I didn't jump off the bridge. I almost wish I had. It would have made a better story, so long as I survived to tell it. What I actually did was step down again and go to Wetherspoons, and order metallic-tasting red wine, and sit there crying into it like a cartoon character, and post something tragic on a Facebook group, and make people worry about me.

I'd love to pretend that it's possible to be cool in crisis – to be edgy, or novelistic, or noble, or really anything but pathetic – but if it is possible to look good losing your mind, I certainly can't do it. I wasn't the girl on the cover of *Prozac Nation* or Angelina Jolie in *Girl, Interrupted*, all collarbones and cigarettes and defiant nihilism. It was just a lot of floundering and thrashing about, afraid to die and afraid to live. I was suffering so much that it consumed everything, and I was relentless in pursuit of relief.

I did try to dial down the long walks after that, which was why I decided to get a bus to the GP appointment. It was the first time I'd ever taken Arthur on a bus. He faced me in his pram while I stood at the bus stop and concentrated very hard on not hurling him or myself into oncoming traffic. As I pushed my weight down on the handlebar, ignoring the sharp tugging sensation in my abdomen, and inexpertly mounted the step onto the bus, I realised that I'd timed our journey badly. We were making our way to the doctors' just as the schools were kicking out.

The bus was rammed with mothers and children of various ages, all yelling and quarrelling and jostling one another. By the time we reached the hill, near the pub and the cottage where Jon and I used to live, somehow there were three pushchairs squeezed on along with my pram. One woman had to fold hers to get past the driver and it dangled awkwardly, half collapsed, from one arm while she clutched a howling toddler in the other. Everyone was flustered; everyone was too warm; no one could get to the doors once their stop came around; and everyone was getting crosser and crosser with everyone else. I couldn't contain it. I couldn't contain my own feelings, let alone a busful of everyone else's.

My heart flapping against my ribcage, I fled, blindly pushing forwards with my pram and apologising universally until the wheels hit pavement, and I tasted fresh air. The low whoosh and growl of passing cars replaced the din inside the bus, and I wept with relief and with shock.

Once I started crying, I couldn't stop. I stood in the street and sobbed great racking, heaving sobs. I've never been an elegant crier. I'd like to gaze pensively out of a window while a single tear slides down my cheek, like in a sad film, but in reality my face goes all puffy and blotchy and there's such a lot of snot. This occasion was particularly undignified, and quite loud. I was trying to rein it in, not because we were in public – I'd forgotten about that entirely – but because I didn't want to frighten Arthur. He looked bemused, almost curious.

As I began to regain composure, I recalled my surroundings. I was still half a mile away from the doctors' surgery, and half a mile uphill at that. Even if I ran – and my chances of running that far were not great – I wasn't going to get there in time for the appointment. I rummaged for my phone, wiping tears and snot off my fingers and onto my cardigan, and in a breathless whimper I told the receptionist that I was running late, but I was on my way.

'How late?'

I had no idea. 'Ten minutes, maybe?'

'You've missed it then,' she said, as bluntly as that, and I had lost my appointment.

I couldn't face making another. It took everything I had to manage myself, moment to moment, and to look after this baby. I couldn't deal with appointments and receptionists and buses as well. I just couldn't. I related my sad tale to one of our pub friends in a long text message and she took it upon herself to call the surgery. I don't know what she said, but almost immediately I learned that I had an appointment the next day. Not only that, but the doctor would be visiting me at home, as if I were the queen or something. I couldn't believe it.

I spent half the night writing a script for this interview, with prompts on my hand in case I drifted off or got

muddled. As soon as the doctor was in front of me, holding a clipboard and pen that she'd produced from a large
leather handbag, I glided smoothly into performance
mode. I spoke clearly and articulately about my bipolar
disorder, the symptoms I was experiencing, and the fact
that I feared for our safety. Fifteen years of patienthood
had prepared me well for this. My words were so precise,
so well selected, surely they couldn't fail to make her
understand.

The words may have been rehearsed but I recited them
naturally, conversationally, those carefully measured rhythms
of speech. I recited them there in my tidy front room, in my
tidy clothes, with my healthy, gurgling baby boy in my lap.
Everything was perfectly controlled and apparently serene. I
smiled small, polite smiles at well-timed moments. I was
coping so beautifully as I told her I wasn't coping.

The coping was part of it. This absurd coping with things
that no one should cope with, this awful resilience, this
instinctive, supplicating response.* It wasn't conscious. It
wasn't a choice. The more distressed I was, the more composed I appeared. This cruel irony had troubled my whole
life. I could be honest, but I could never be transparent. I
could ask for help, and I could be oh-so-very clear and
specific about how bad things were, but I could never show
anyone what I was like when I was alone. I was surrounded
by kind people who cared for me, but they could never get
near me when I needed them most. I could never bridge
that vast chasm between my external presentation and my
internal reality, which was then mirrored in the chasm

---

* In groping for language to describe this experience, I've benefited from
online conversations with my friend Heather Cobb, and from her tweets.

between me and everyone else. At best, it was lonely, and at worst, it was dangerous.

The doctor's tone was brisk and amiable. 'I'll write to your psychiatrist,' she said, 'but you might find it's nothing a good night's sleep won't sort out.'

I asked how long it would take for Dr Freyman to receive her letter. 'It's just . . . I think it might be a bit more urgent than that?'

'Oh, not more than two or three weeks,' she said. 'I'll fax it.'

My next memory is of late that night in the waiting area at A & E, Arthur asleep in his car seat and Jon scrolling robotically through his phone. I watched his fingers swipe, swipe, swipe so fast he couldn't possibly be taking anything in. Eventually we were shown to a small room with framed pictures on the walls, padded chairs, and a box of tissues on the table. This was the room where they broke bad news. I had been in that room before, right before they carted me off to the bin in an ambulance. The room did not bode well.

The doctor who joined us there was one I hadn't met. I think he was a psychiatrist. Presumably he had a name. Everything he said to me in the first few minutes was drowned out by the fact that he looked and sounded exactly like the actor Michael Caine. It was uncanny. In other circumstances, I don't think I could have resisted commenting but it's just as well that I didn't. He must get it all the time. His friends must be constantly setting him up to say, 'You were only supposed to blow the bloody doors off.'[2]

It took me a little while to adjust to undergoing a psychiatric assessment with Michael Caine but actually, he was wonderful. I don't know if he'd had better training or if he just had better instincts, but I said and did pretty much exactly what I'd said and done with the GP twelve hours earlier, and he took me completely seriously. He said that we had done the right thing in coming to hospital, and that I needed to go to a psychiatric mother and baby unit (known as an MBU), where I could get the specialist help that I needed and stay with my baby.

But we were back to clinical pathways. Michael Caine didn't have the power to send me to an MBU himself. He could only arrange for me to see Dr Freyman at the community mental health service first thing in the morning. He wrote a note recommending that I should be admitted to an MBU, with Arthur, as soon as possible.

So began a week of pass-the-parcel, in which I was the parcel. At each appointment, someone unpacked me, surveyed my component parts, and packaged me up again to ship to the next person. Everyone agreed that I should go into an MBU, but no one had the power to send me there. Everyone believed that the next person they sent me to would be the one to make the necessary arrangements. From Michael Caine I went to Dr Freyman; from Dr Freyman I was shunted to the home treatment team, a crisis service who send someone to visit you at home each day. The first person who came couldn't do the referral, but then someone else could. We lived that week on a knife edge.

News came that Arthur and I were to be admitted at the mother and baby unit in Winchester, fifty miles away. We decided that Jon would go back to Southampton and stay with his parents, so that he would be nearer and more able to visit. We would have to shut up our home indefinitely. April the cat would take an extended holiday. That one was a guilty relief: she was livid that I'd brought this miniature screaming human into her queendom and would seek me out so that she could pointedly sit with her back to me.

I found someone to take her. I begged us a lift to Winchester. I emptied the fridge. Hayley came over and helped me to pack, as I flitted from room to room fretting that I had too much stuff but also that I definitely needed all of it: babygros, nappies, wipes, changing mat, bottles, formula powder, formula prep machine, muslins, bibs, a notebook for me to write in, ideally some clothes for me as well . . . It seems bizarre that I oversaw this whole operation while on suicide watch, but I did. I was steeled to hold myself together, to hold everything together, until we were safe. At least, I hoped we'd be safe.

Melbury Lodge

Can't he see what happens
when words confront the truth?
They scatter like rats.

Polly Clark, 'Dora'[1]

April 2014

I t didn't look like a hospital, certainly not like the eerie,
dilapidated psychiatric ward I'd come to know so well.
I stepped into Melbury Lodge and saw cream walls, cream
carpets, and a framed print of Gustav Klimt's painting of a
mother and child sleeping, rosy-cheeked, her corn-
coloured hair dotted with tiny flowers.

A nurse with curly grey hair had answered the door and
introduced herself as Esther. We all bundled in: me and Jon,
little Arthur still asleep in his car seat, and our friend Tom,
who had driven us all the way to Winchester. Esther led us
to a bedroom – not a dormitory, I noted, but my own
bedroom – with an ensuite bathroom, proper duvet on
a proper bed, chest of drawers, full-sized wooden cot,
and tub-shaped armchair in brown leather. The mother

and baby unit had ten of these bedrooms, all along one corridor.

When Esther gave us the tour, I saw there was also a café-style kitchen and dining area; a milk kitchen for the babies' formula; a lounge with sofas and television; a nursery with toys, playmats, and smaller cots; an outdoor courtyard; a laundry room; a few other smaller rooms for meetings or individual therapy; and a spirituality or faith room. There were other mums and babies around, mental health nurses, and nursery nurses on hand to help with baby care. On a typical day, Esther explained, you would look after your baby, perhaps see a psychiatrist or psychologist, or attend a group session, and you might do a group activity such as baby massage or baking. You could go into town once you had the okay to do so from the doctor, and you could pop to the hospital Costa.

I don't know what I had anticipated, but it wasn't this. I half suspected it was all an elaborate trick, that once Jon and Tom had left and the door closed behind them, someone would pull back a curtain to reveal the *actual* mother and baby unit. Or perhaps, like at Maplewood, the pleasant surroundings would be an ironic backdrop for many subtle and not-so-subtle cruelties.

We settled back in my bedroom and Esther brought mugs of tea and biscuits on a plate. The tea was scalding hot, but I drank it straight away, felt it hurt as it went down my throat and into my chest. Esther seemed in no hurry for Jon and Tom to leave. They sipped their tea. I don't know what we talked about. Then, of course, it was time for them to get back in the car and on the motorway, while Arthur and I remained behind.

I felt a sudden wild stab of panic. Please, I wanted to say.

Please don't leave me here. Please don't leave me here with the baby.

I didn't say that because it wouldn't be fair. Whatever was going to happen to us here was going to happen.

'I'll be back tomorrow evening,' said Jon, although he knew that I knew that.

Esther showed them out while I sat on the bed, staring at the carpet.

I eyed her warily as she returned. She was talking to me, but I was drifting again, floating in that clouded, billowy place between past and present, between real and make-believe.

She seemed to be saying, 'Can I hug you?'

'I'm sorry, what?'

'Would you like a hug?'

'Um, okay?'

I flinched and stiffened as Esther put her arms around me, my own arms like rods at my side. She squeezed me briefly and, confused and incredulous as I was to be hugged by a nurse in this way, I felt the care that came with the gesture. It was a sense that, deranged as I might be, I was not beyond hugs, or tea and biscuits, or fellow feeling from someone who was sane.

'I'll let you get settled,' she said. 'Come and find me if you need anything.'

Much like when we moved house and April spent half a day at the back of the wardrobe, I needed that time to be alone in a small space, to gather my courage. Eventually, like April, I put my nose around the door and peered out, then crept gingerly across the carpet to scout what might be lurking beyond.

There was a board on the wall with rectangular

photographs of each member of staff and their name and job title written underneath, like a giant game of Guess Who?. I felt an urge to flick them with my fingernail, make them fold down with a clatter. I found Esther's face. She could stay upright. I stood there a while, scanning the photos, asking each of them silently, So I've placed myself and my baby in your hands. Who are you, then?

One mugshot caught my eye: a man with an enormous dark moustache. His label named him as Dr Alain Gregoire, consultant psychiatrist. French, apparently. I said his name to myself in an exaggerated French accent, like Pepé Le Pew.

That evening, I took up the notebook I'd packed, found a pen, and began to write:

5 *April 2014*

Dearest Arthur,

Here we are at the mother and baby unit in Winchester. Little one, this is not the start I envisaged for you. I look back at my life, bouncing between hospitalisations, and I know that this has to change, for your sake. So I'm here and I'm fighting for whatever help is going to sort me out. I'm trying to ignore the fear, the one in four, that you may have inherited this disease. In my less optimistic moments, I see it as a life sentence at best and a death sentence at worst. I don't want your life to look like this. Sometimes I wonder if it was selfish of me to have you. Nor do I want you to be scarred by having a mad mother. I will keep trying to fix this, I promise you.

In spite of everything, I do feel hopeful. It's so lovely here. The staff are excellent. Even if we can't get me sorted, it was worth uprooting our little family and coming here.

I've just handed you over for the night. It was a wrench, but I know you're in really good hands. I briefed them extensively about your little quirks. They will probably do a better job than I would, and I will be a more competent mother for the sleep. I can't imagine any more what it will be like to sleep.

Speaking of sleep, I hope to soon get on with it.

I love you, little one. I'm not sorry I brought us here. I will always fight for you and for our family. May you always know that your mum would do anything.

I wrote Arthur a letter every day for the first few weeks we were there, then more sporadically, trailing off as we began to look to going home. I don't know why I decided to write letters to someone who couldn't read and was right there beside me. I don't know if he'll want to read them one day. But I am glad that I wrote them. I'm glad to have the record. The letters are testament to the fact that I loved him from the start. I loved him before it felt like love.

As I write this chapter, it's the first time I've revisited that notebook. The thin blue biro I'd picked up somewhere makes my handwriting look particularly round and childish on the lined pages. It occurs to me how young I was for twenty-six, and how hard I was trying, all the time. The letters circle endlessly around my dilemma, that I simply didn't know what to do to make myself sane. It's not that the motivation wasn't there before. I was suffering and very motivated to fix that. I was desperate, in fact. I'd seen all these mental health professionals and was falling over myself to enable them to reach me, to help me. But the stakes were so much higher once Arthur was here. It was imperative that my life change radically, and quickly. And I didn't have the first idea how to make that happen.

After I finished that first letter, I did sleep. I woke at one and tiptoed along the shadowy corridor, round to the nursery, hovering there while Arthur slept among the other babies. Having been ushered back to bed, I fell asleep again at three. I'd set an alarm for eight but rose only briefly, then slept on through most of the day, and all the next night, and most of the following day as well.

My parents came to visit, and Arthur beamed at them, enchanting as ever. Again, I slept all night and most of the next day. All that oblivion did seem to reboot my brain somewhat and I began to feel ... not better, exactly, but groping towards it. I was still in two minds about whether growing up without me would be better or worse for Arthur than growing up with me. For over a decade I had feared that I was a lost cause, but it wasn't about that. My centre of gravity had shifted: it was all about protecting him, mentally as much as physically. Protecting him even from myself.

A psychiatric hospital is its own world, a microcosm, and you shrink to fit. The world outside doesn't quite cease to exist, but it becomes distant, a backdrop for the really important issues, like when will you be able to catch a washing machine empty or persuade someone to chaperone you to Costa. And of course, when will you see the psychiatrist. It's the psychiatrist who decides what you can and can't do, where you can and can't go, how closely you must be watched and what medication you must take. Queries about diagnostic labels or side effects, petitions, requests for leave ... everything gets saved up for that one weekly interview.

When my turn came to sit down with Dr Gregoire, I was more than ready. I knew the drill. You follow a stranger into a small room. There are two or three chairs and a low table with a strategically placed box of tissues. The stranger wears an NHS lanyard and holds a clipboard with printed information about you that's too small to read from where you're sitting. Handwritten notes will be added as you talk. The psychiatrist will open with something along the lines of: 'You're here. Oh dear. You've had a manic episode / depressed episode / mixed episode [delete as appropriate]. We'll increase your medication.' There's not much else to say.

The safest bet is to keep that conversation as uncomplicated as possible. Agree with everything the psychiatrist says. Ask one or two questions so that he knows you're engaging with him and that you defer to his expertise. Be sure to appear grateful. In between encounters, keep your head down and stay out of everyone's way. Everything that happens will be reported back.

As I followed Dr Gregoire into that small room with its chairs and low table and tissues, I didn't dare to hope for anything else.

He sat down, revealing brightly coloured, zanily patterned socks. Then he put the papers he was holding to one side and leaned forward, resting his elbows on his knees.

'So, Laura, would you like to tell me about what's brought you here?'

'Um, I think I might have postnatal PTSD.' I began to rattle off my symptoms, describing in turn the flashbacks, intrusive thoughts, anxiety . . . I reduced the horror of the past six weeks to a checklist, as I thought was required. I moved on to talk about feeling suicidal, as that was technically the reason we'd been admitted to hospital, outlining that in my usual dispassionate style. But I was increasingly thrown by his blue-grey eyes fixed on me behind his glasses, and the fact that he was listening intently to every word I said.

'It does sound like you've had a very difficult, very frightening time of it over the last few weeks.'

'Yeah.' I was a little irritated that he seemed to be going off script already. Stating the obvious, I thought. Really, it was just that I didn't want to go there. I didn't want to acknowledge that I was frightened. I didn't want to look that one in the face any more than I wanted to look at him. I didn't want to feel it, any of it. I certainly didn't want him to see it.

I steered us back on course: 'Do you think I have PTSD?'

'Well, PTSD isn't typically diagnosed until six months after the event, but certainly I'd say it sounds like the trauma around Arthur's birth has really affected you.'

I said nothing.

'This might be difficult to answer and don't worry if you don't want to, but have any other things happened which could be described as traumatic – in your childhood, perhaps?'

I didn't know what to say. Of course other things had happened. I'd spent more than half my life as a fully paid-up mentalist, for one. It wasn't so much skeletons in the closet as the entire basement being a plague pit with the tibias and toe bones of a hundred diseased unfortunates squeezing up through the floorboards.

I was caught between the need to be seen to do exactly as I was told, and the urge to get as far away from Dr Gregoire and his kind, listening face as humanly possible. I heard myself recounting a list of traumatic and potentially traumatic events in chronological order. It sounded comical, so completely blasé. As if I could trump the indifference I was expecting with my own indifference. As if these were separate events that I experienced one at a time, one after another, all firmly past tense. Or as if I never experienced them at all. I wasn't lying, but I may as well have been.

He let me finish, and quickly said, 'I don't need to know the details. People who experience the kinds of things that you're describing often also tell me that they've had some difficult experiences in childhood, and it sounds like that's been the case for you too. But you really don't need to tell me the details.'

In that moment, I did want to tell him – not the stupid, ambiguous details of all the stupid, ambiguous things that had happened. Not my symptoms either. I wanted to tell him how it felt. How it feels. I wanted to tell him to sit tight and listen, because this happened. I lived it. I was still living it, and I needed someone to know.

I needed someone to know that I didn't know any more what was within me and what was without. That since Arthur was born, all the things that had ever happened in my life had fractured into a kaleidoscope, and no one had warned me about that, or I wouldn't have had him. That I was perpetually caught between wanting to bury it all deep in the woods in the middle of the night so that no one would ever, ever find it or me, and wanting to scream everything from the rooftops, to seize someone, anyone, and make them see. And that ambivalence, the both-at-once, made it unbearable to be near anyone, because I was afraid that I might just start blurting it all out, and if I started talking about these things, I would howl and howl and I would never stop.

And I was back behind a wooden door with a frosted glass panel and all I could see was the blurred outline of Jon walking away.

I heard screams and realised that they were my own.

The candles along the mantlepiece were flickering and struggling as if fighting for their lives.

The side of the birth pool slammed into my body, and the body of a huge male nurse slammed into my body, and the floor, glittering, rose to meet me.

Dr Gregoire sounded as if he were underwater. I scratched at my thigh with my fingernail and made an effort to listen.

He said, 'I think you might have something called complex PTSD.'

A diagnosis! Thank fuck. We were back on course. If I got another diagnosis, maybe I would understand how to fix this, and I could not be mad any more and be a good mum to Arthur.

Dr Gregoire said that the problems I was having, and that I'd had to varying degrees for so many years, sounded like a reaction to childhood trauma – or adversity, which might be a better term. There are some things that can have a long-term impact on us if we experience them as a child, an impact which lasts into our adult life. And this crisis, after a traumatic birth, was completely understandable: trauma reawakens trauma.

There was an instinctive gut feeling of rightness about this, but it didn't quite add up. If any of the events and circumstances I'd listed constituted trauma that had made me the way I was, why wasn't there a 'before' time – a time when I was like everybody else? I couldn't recall such a time. Everything just gradually got worse. It was a dripping tap that became a flood, a snowball rolled until it caused an eclipse. And much of the textbook trauma happened after my eighteenth birthday, so not in my childhood at all.

I made this point, careful to phrase it as a question so that it would be read as my consulting an expert rather than a challenge to authority. 'If complex PTSD is something that develops in childhood, when's the cut-off for that?'

He seemed comfortable – pleased, even – that I wanted to critique his idea and start a dialogue about it.

'Well, research shows that actually our brains are developing right up to the age of twenty-five – and beyond.'

'I'm twenty-six. All right. So, what about bipolar? Am I not bipolar after all?'

'I don't know. You might be, or you might not. But I suspect the main issue, in terms of what's going on for you right now, could well be complex PTSD.'

The suggestion that bipolar could have been a misdiagnosis all along was too much to contemplate. It was such a huge part of who I understood myself to be. And all those drugs, all those side effects ... I willed Dr Gregoire back into focus.

He was saying that, with complex PTSD, emotions can

change rapidly and intensely, and that can be mistaken for bipolar disorder. If we learn that the world is dangerous, and that people are dangerous, and that any little thing could signal danger – the sound of footsteps, or a door opening, or the way someone looks at us – those tiny, commonplace signals can make us intensely anxious. And, if we've learned and absorbed this in such a programmed way, we don't necessarily recognise what's set us off and why, and so we get these sudden changes in mood. They're part of watching out for danger.

Would that make you elated, though? I wondered. Excitable? I'd always thought that my manic moods seemed to have more to do with lack of sleep than anything else. I'd been told that I couldn't sleep because I was manic, but I was beginning to wonder if I became manic because I couldn't sleep.

Dr Gregoire continued, 'And if we have intrusive memories and thoughts, they can be so vivid that we might call them visions or voices, and of course that gets psychiatrists really excited.'

I thought of Dr Haslam and how, when I told him about my voices, he *had* genuinely seemed excited. Then he sent me to Maplewood.

The voices had never fully gone away, but I'd stopped calling them voices because it made people freak out, or, like Dr Pinhead, they simply didn't believe me. Anyway, they weren't exactly voices. I didn't know the word for what they were. I recognised them, for the first time, in what Dr Gregoire called 'non-psychotic voices' – because it's not like hearing them through your ears. They're clearly and intensely inside your head.

I was beginning to think he had got the measure of me,

and he was still going, as I queried or affirmed what he was saying by turns.

'You know, children, when they're trapped in unbearable situations and can't physically get away, have this amazing capacity to just mentally get away and shut off. They build fantasy worlds. And if that becomes embedded as a technique for protecting themselves, that's what we call dissociation.'

I didn't tell him about the wizard in my nan's shower. Or about that whole parallel universe, heavily borrowed from *The Magician's Nephew* by C. S. Lewis, where I went when I sat in the playground with my coat over my head. I didn't mention Bethany Fleamarket and Jane Hunt and One-Legged Margaret, or any of my ghost pals, or Sunflower, my imaginary horse. I didn't describe the pressure to outgrow all of that, or how suppressing it and hiding it by turns had twisted everything into knots. I could feel it under my fingernails, clinging on to what was being ripped from my grasp. I knew that it was normal for children to enjoy imaginative play, and I knew that the way I did it wasn't normal. It was too real, too essential. Perhaps I didn't need to tell him any of that because he said it for me.

'Laura, would you like to take a break?'

'No, no, sorry. What did you say?'

'I was just saying about dissociation, that it's a very helpful way of dealing with trauma, but not a helpful way of leading your life.'

Fair, I suppose.

Unnerving as it was that Dr Gregoire seemed to know all these things about me that I'd never told anyone, I was starting to feel more at ease. There was something disarming and rather likable about the conviction with which he spoke. This felt like a proper conversation, in which I could interrogate his theory and raise issues with it as they occurred to me.

'What you're describing as complex PTSD,' I said, 'sounds a lot like what I've read about borderline personality disorder. They decided I had that – well, they said it was *emerging* BPD, because I was fifteen and not an adult yet – when I was in hospital the first time. Do you think they were right?'

'Well, I certainly don't believe that you have a disorder of your personality. To me that seems like a nonsensical way of labelling people and understanding their problems. But the term personality disorder is very commonly used, even though we've known for decades that so-called borderline personality disorder has a powerful association with trauma in childhood. Complex PTSD is a much more accurate way of understanding these difficulties. These are very, very understandable reactions to childhood adversity. Laura, you must understand that you are a hero. You are an extraordinary survivor.'

I stared hard at his socks. I couldn't see that continuing to exist was much of an achievement. Bare minimum, arguably. And in fact, I had tried to off myself more than once: my survival was more down to my own cack-handedness and ignorance of human anatomy than anything else.

'You've got this far in your life. You've found ways of tackling it, but maybe, particularly now, these ways that you've managed to tick away with are particularly difficult and unhelpful because you have Arthur. So, let's see if we can actually make things better.'

I felt a great surge of hope, all bells ringing and angels singing, as Dr Gregoire talked about the emotional coping-skills course at the mother and baby unit, and after that, something called dialectical behaviour therapy, or DBT. Perhaps I didn't always have to feel this way. The raw skinlessness of it, the splintering hurt, and all the stupid, desperate ways I would relieve that hurt like cutting myself or mapping out how I would end my life – there really could be a time after all that and a version of me without it. Perhaps this was the turning point. Perhaps I really could be the mum that Arthur needed.

'Sign me up,' I said.

———

Everything I thought I knew about myself was suddenly up for debate. I left Arthur in the nursery, took myself off to my bedroom, and firmly closed the door. Headphones on, I started pacing so that I could begin to process all this new information.

What Dr Gregoire had said felt right. It felt like when the name of a book or a song or a person has been on the tip of your tongue for weeks, driving you spare, and you reach and reach but can't quite grasp it, and everyone you ask looks at you blankly. Then one day someone says, 'Oh! You mean——?' There it was all along.

And yet, the idea of my having complex PTSD created a tangled, knotty discomfort. It implied all sorts of things about my upbringing, about my family, and none of them seemed fair. I didn't like the blame hovering in the background. I had a lovely childhood in lots of ways. I was always warm, and fed, and cared for. Rather spoilt, in fact.

Who was I, with my ordinary life and ordinary misery, to claim complex PTSD? Some non-ideal things had happened, but non-ideal things happened to everyone. I'd had a better time – in mental health services and in life generally – than most people. I couldn't ignore or deny the great, thundering, unfair advantages that carried me through it all: being educated, having enough money, a good home, a loving family ... I felt that admitting I'd been so badly wounded, and arguably by nothing much, amounted to a snivelling self-pity deserving only of contempt. Get over yourself, I thought.

In fact, the voice I heard was Mrs Wentworth, echoing down the years: 'Normal life isn't exciting enough for you, is it? You have to glam it up a bit. You're a drama queen. Don't you realise how lucky you are?'

'And how fucking convenient,' added every other inner voice, 'to be handed a narrative that paints you not only as a victim, but – get this – as the heroine of the piece, when all you've done is cry and hurt yourself and create trouble for people who love you. No wonder you think this is your eureka moment. It's your get-out card for having to take responsibility.'

I realised, as I was pacing up and down to Katy Perry – who wouldn't have been my first choice, or even my fiftieth, but was on the iPod I'd borrowed ahead of going into hospital – that I was going to have to put these reservations aside.

I wanted the therapy. I wanted the chance so badly. I wanted to be Arthur's mum.

I seized the notebook of letters and began to write:

I saw the consultant today and he gave me something of a new perspective ... His diagnosis: what is sometimes called borderline personality disorder but he calls 'complex PTSD'.

He says it's a response to childhood trauma. He called me a survivor and a hero and made me embarrassed. But I do think he made a lot of sense. The plan is this coping-skills course while I'm here and, hopefully, dialectical behaviour therapy once we go home. I don't know if it will help but I will give it my all for you. Anything is worth trying.

Homecoming

sweet child
this is not an undoing
but a remaking
measured on a pattern
older than time

Lulu Allison, *Salt Lick*[1]

April to May 2014

Later that week, I tried having Arthur sleep in my room for the first time since we came to Melbury Lodge. The wooden cot seemed huge, and he was terrifyingly tiny inside it, so instead I wheeled his crib from the nursery along the corridor and parked it next to my bed. I lay there past midnight, the vilest little video montage of smothering him with my pillow playing on a loop as he slept peacefully beside me.

When I couldn't take it any more, I fled the room and sat hunched on the carpet just outside the door. A nurse offered lorazepam to calm me down and help me sleep, but I was afraid that if I took it, I might not wake to tend to

Arthur. He would be hungry, stranded in an unfamiliar place, powerless to do anything to help himself, kicking his little legs and howling desperation into the dark ... After repeated reassurances, I took the lorazepam and went back to bed.

My limbs were heavy against the mattress. It was as if I had smothered myself with that pillow, but there was still something flailing at the core of me. I distracted myself by scrolling through Facebook, until I saw that someone had posted something jokey about childbirth on one of the mum groups. Memories seized me like a marionette. One by one, they shook me and flung me down, discarded and broken on the bedsheets. It was too dark and still in that room, too much space for past and future events to leap in and take over. I had some more lorazepam, and wheeled Arthur back to the nursery.

What sort of mother couldn't be in a room with her own child? I panicked about that for a while, alone amid the grey-black silhouettes of the furniture, then I was standing in the corridor in my nightie like a toddler out of bed for the umpteenth time. No more lorazepam was going, so I had some zopiclone instead, and I left my door ajar, afraid of the dark for the first time in my life. I needed to look at things to stave off the scenes of birth–death and baby murder that my mind imprinted onto every blank canvas.

Back in bed once more, I still couldn't sleep, and with the door half open there was enough light to write.

I don't know why I picked now to grieve for everything that's gone wrong in my life. I am just so ... ravaged. The places I've been. The things that were done to my body. And this isn't the first time I've failed to hold it together on the floor of a psychiatric ward. Is it the last? I couldn't bear for your life to look like mine. I am so sorry. Sometimes I wish I could transport you away from all of this, from me.

Three days later, we tried again. I don't recall that attempt at all, but I wrote, '*I kept falling asleep while feeding you, so I reluctantly handed you over again . . . I swear I had more to say but it's gone now.*'

Another three days and I managed it: Arthur stayed in my room all night. The second tongue-tie snip had worked its magic and he slept nine and a half hours straight through.

'*If only I had too,*' I noted wryly. I'd spent that night perched on the end of the bed, watching Arthur's chest rise and fall.

When I next saw Dr Gregoire, he wanted to put me back on quetiapine – a tiny dose, he assured me, nothing like what I was on in my teens – just to take the edge off so that I wouldn't be watching Arthur all night. I agreed, because old habits die hard, but later I hid the pill in my cheek and then flushed it down the toilet. I had to stay vigilant in case Arthur needed me.

It was a constant weighing up: my needs versus his. Later, I began to relish finding creative ways to get everyone's conflicting needs met simultaneously. I became more resourceful and more adaptable than I ever gave myself credit for at the time. But in those early months, I was too shattered, too precariously held together, to have that mental bend and flex. The idea of Arthur suffering was so real and ever-present.

Meanwhile, I'd started attending the emotional coping-skills course. It was a sort of DBT-lite: weekly group sessions in which we would learn coping strategies drawn from dialectical behaviour therapy. I'd like to say that I was cool and nonchalant during these sessions, or that I challenged individualistic approaches to mental health that neglect societal and structural factors, but the truth is I was embarrassingly keen. Any question posed to the group and my hand would shoot up. 'Pick me, Miss, oooh pick me! I know the answer!'

I wasn't quite as bad as that, but almost.

At the beginning of every session, there was a review of the homework. Everyone else either hadn't done it or they'd had a half-hearted stab at it in the twenty minutes before we went in, but I'd done everything, and I'd made up extra for myself as well. I handwrote whole essays assessing my own competence at 'distress tolerance' and 'radical acceptance' and utilising the 'DEAR MAN' acronym strategy for effective communication. I dutifully suppressed my longing to aim a bit higher than simply not inconveniencing others with my soul-eating distress. I suppressed the view that some things are and should be straight-up unacceptable, and that acronyms are annoying. This was for Arthur, and I was going to change myself to become the absolute most skilled at emotional coping for ever, for his sake.

Esther welcomed my enthusiasm. We had serious one-to-ones in which she coached me on the techniques, recommended books, and even laminated printed cards with reminders for me to keep. I loved her for her commitment to 'The Skills' and to my proficiency at employing them. We were determined that I would become so adept while I was in hospital that it would tide me over until I started the full DBT course, and that I would arrive with a head start. '*It goes on for a year,*' I wrote, '*and sounds properly hardcore.*' I had no idea how I would find the time or childcare for multiple sessions a week over such a long period, but if someone was willing to put that much into me, I was going to find a way.

'MY SUBJECTIVE FEELINGS DO NOT DETERMINE ALL OF REALITY FOREVER,' I scrawled in huge letters, and Blu-Tacked it above my bed.

There was one problem with my new mad skills, and that was that they didn't work. As I stilled myself and focused on my breathing, all was, initially, fine – but then I found that I couldn't breathe unless I was consciously thinking about it, and how the hell was I going to switch myself back to the automatic breathing setting, because this was exhausting, and my chest was tired and my brain was tired, and my chest felt tight and my head was aching, but I must keep going, because if I didn't breathe I would actually die, and what if I was stuck like this, and oh god . . .

As for self-care activities, I could only hope that as I persevered, I would begin to dislike them less. Colouring-in bored me. It felt infantilising. Hand cream was, well, handy, in that it was useful after washing up so many baby bottles, but that was all. Bringing it out when I felt suicidal just left me suicidal with greasy hands. Chocolate was delicious, granted, but not beneficial in the quantities required to snack myself sane. Most of all, none of these strategies or activities or hacks ever actually made me any less upset.

It must be me, I thought, awkward and perverse and complicated, as usual. I resolved to try harder. I had to believe that if I tried hard enough for long enough, I would learn how to be like everyone else. So, I sat with my colouring pencils in the nursery or the lounge, scowling at a mandala and slamming every door in my head on how much better it would feel to just jam the sharpened pencil into my thigh. If colouring and breathing and acronyms were the path to serenity, so be it. I certainly wasn't going to acknowledge that I was struggling with 'The Skills', even to myself. There was too much riding on them. And I was so eager to please Esther with my progress that it was easy to lie a little and not really notice.

I was a polite, unmemorable patient. It wasn't that I wanted or needed to be, but over the years I'd learned that was the safest course and it had become my default. If I was going to lose my shit, I took myself away and did that in private. I went to my hospital bedroom and closed the door firmly behind me.

Alone in that little room, I absorbed the shock of Arthur's birth and everything that had happened. It was there that I felt, fully for the first time, how wrecked I was, how smashed against the rocks. It was there that I fell apart, splinters on the waves of my own grief. It hit me over and over, this hard tide, and all I could do was weep as it kept coming.

I had been cut open with a scalpel. A stranger's gloved hands rummaged inside my abdomen. There was groping and feeling and pulling in the white-grey light, stale and sterile. My child was a red blur, a smudge of blood, a streaky setting sun. He crossed the sky above me and was gone. He could have died. I could have died. The doctors and midwives had saved our lives and here we were, intact. I knew that we were lucky, but I couldn't summon the gratitude I was supposed to feel. I could never be vast enough to contain the aching void between everything I had hoped for, for myself and most of all for Arthur, and what had happened. I could never contain that operating theatre and its instruments, its gowned figures. I had failed Arthur. I failed at being his mum before I even began.

I crumpled on the carpet, and then I washed my face and returned to smile and eat lunch and do laundry. It became almost routine.

As days and weeks passed, my death wish receded like the tide. The intrusive thoughts and memories still washed around me, but I wasn't drowning in them any more. I slept. I left Arthur in the nursery. I carried him around with me and read him *Room on the Broom*. The bleeding that was or wasn't a period got shallower, trailed off, and finally stopped altogether.

Annette reappeared for my discharge meeting. Jon and I exchanged the briefest of glances as she told Dr Gregoire and Esther all about the 'intensive support' I would have from the community mental health service once we were home. I couldn't think of anything worse, or indeed anything less likely, but there was no point in saying so. There was nothing Dr Gregoire could do about what happened at a different service in a different part of the country. At least he wouldn't know. It wasn't as if I were ever going to see him again. He smiled at me across the room, creases in the corners of his eyes. I smiled back.

A referral for DBT was being arranged, and people around me spoke in warm, hopeful voices. I felt hopeful too. I felt like I'd stepped through a doorway. I had a new diagnosis, a new framework for understanding my own particular genre of madness, and a plan was in place, not just to mitigate but to actually remedy it. This was a new story for my life, one with a happier ending.

Most of all, I had been believed. Not once, at Melbury Lodge, had anyone ever made me feel that I shouldn't be there. No one had implied that I was making it up or making a fuss. It was as if I'd had the second chance I dreamed of after Maplewood, and it was a redemption of sorts, to go into hospital and be treated kindly while I was there. I had spent my whole life saying, 'It hurts. Please believe me.' And I had finally been heard.

I left the mother and baby unit a little wiser and a lot less wretched than when I arrived. Esther cried when I said goodbye. I cried too. Then I pushed Arthur's pram to the train station with Jon at my side, both of us quiet and thoughtful.

Melbury Lodge saved my life. It wasn't the drugs that they gave me, or the emotional coping-skills course, or the presence of the nurses, or even the conversations with Dr Gregoire. More than anything, I needed a safe place to confront everything that had happened. Only once I stared down those facts, and assimilated them, would I be ready to meet my baby. That hospital bedroom was where I began to seek and gather all the parts of myself that had scattered across the ocean of birth. Only I could do that, and I needed to do it alone. I needed to leave Arthur in the nursery sometimes so that I didn't have to leave him altogether. And I needed the knives out of reach while I felt it all, because I would so rather not have felt it.

—

The day before Arthur turned three months old, something strange and wonderful happened. It was early morning. Jon had already left for work. I was in the attic room, dozing as soft new light crept in and pooled on the crumpled bedsheets. Arthur began to stir in the Moses basket beside me, kicking off his blanket in the late-spring warmth. I sat up and watched him.

His arms were folded above his head in mirror image of

his still-froggy legs. His skin was plump and creamy, his elbows creased. With his head to one side, he slept posed like a strongman, like a champion. He twitched a little, turned his head towards me and opened his eyes – so blue, the bluest eyes I've ever seen – and they lit up with recognition as he saw me.

'Good morning,' I said. He gurgled a greeting and kicked his legs happily, so obviously delighted to find himself there, with me.

I tucked my hands beneath his arms and lifted him onto my pillow, and that was when I saw him, actually *saw* him for the first time – my loving, sociable, happy baby boy. Somehow it had completely escaped my notice that I had a son. I hadn't realised that this was the same baby I'd carried and dreamed of for nine long months. Here he was. Here. This was Arthur. Something in me met something in him and found its place, like a homing instinct, swift and true. There was your 'rush of love'.

'Holy shit, I made a person,' I breathed. 'Hello, Arthur.'

He beamed at me, and I realised that every other love I'd ever known had only skipped across the surface of what it is to love. To protect him, I would quite cheerfully throw anyone else into a volcano. I would die in a heartbeat. I would submit to anything. This love was so weighty I'd feel crushed by it at times. It would bring tears to my eyes as I held him drifting off to sleep.

I am so lucky to be his mum. The day he was born, the universe rearranged itself around him. And what an honour – utterly unasked for, unthought of – to be loved so straightforwardly, and to be someone's refuge, first port of call. This love is alive, ever growing, ever shifting, and it has fundamentally altered me.

I realised, then, what I did not even know I had doubted: you do not have to breastfeed to bond with your baby. You don't have to give birth in a bath of rose petals while Tibetan monks chant blessings around you. Nothing has to go to plan, nothing at all. You don't have to wear your child in a sling or sleep with them in your bed, or anything else that my inner earth mother longed for and was denied. You don't even have to be particularly sane. You just have to love them, to cultivate the freedom to feel that love and to show it.

I will never be able to give birth in the way that I'd hoped, but I could parent that way: instinctively, intuitively, trusting my body to know what to do. Every time I scooped him up into my arms, every time I carried him on my hip, every time I heard that cry in the darkness and went to him. We were not quite separate, not quite two people, not yet. I would notice it most in his absence: unthinkingly pushing a trolley back and forth in the supermarket queue, crossing the road and reaching down for a little hand that was at home. I'd never been so unselfconscious.

Sometimes love is a rush, and sometimes it's a steady climb. I think that's true of healing as well. As I loved and was loved, something began to shift in the way that I am with myself, how I fuel and affirm and steady myself. I wasn't cured, far from it, but the direction of travel had changed, even if it would take me a few years to notice. In the loving and tending, in the watchful waiting, the feeding and rocking and shushing and responding, I began to reconnect with my own body, to feel what it felt and know what it knew. To tune into Arthur was to tune into myself, to feel the thrumming of my body and mind, to return home.

four

A Pink Toothbrush

... no one is finally dead until the ripples they cause in the world die away – until the clock he wound up winds down, until the wine she made has finished its ferment, until the crop they planted is harvested. The span of someone's life, they say, is only the core of their actual existence.

Terry Pratchett, *Reaper Man*[1]

Early summer 2014

I sat in the bright June sunshine and picked at blades of grass with my fingers. The bus timetable had dictated that I arrive half an hour early or ten minutes late, so I'd opted for the former. I thought best to avoid prolonging my stint in the waiting room and instead find somewhere outdoors on the hospital grounds, somewhere free of leaflets and Blu-Tack-speckled walls.

I had not, in fact, been referred for therapy. Instead, I had to see a psychiatrist at the community mental health service who would assess me and decide whether to refer me to the personality disorder service. That was where the DBT happened. The landscape was always shifting like this, but I was used to it, so I accepted the news without complaint, boarded my too-early bus, and found a sunny spot to settle down.

I wasn't thinking about the assessment, or therapy, or my personality and its potential disorders. I was trying to wrap my head around weaning. The thing about babies – and children, actually – is that they're always with you, even when they aren't. You can leave them with someone else and take a bus and go elsewhere, but then you can't stop thinking about them. That's the relentlessness of it.

I'd stopped at Sainsbury's on my way and bought four different boxes of baby porridge, although I was also minded to try 'baby-led weaning', a rather grand term for giving them some food and letting them get on with it. We might as well throw everything at the wall and see what sticks. Hopefully Arthur wouldn't take that too literally.

I studied the boxes. They all claimed to be suitable 'from four to six months', while everything else I'd read advised that weaning should start at six months, or when baby can sit up unassisted. Which, though? Arthur couldn't sit totally unassisted – he would wobble and sway like a little Weeble and eventually topple sideways – but he was quite happy strapped into a highchair. Did that count? I would compare notes with Hayley. She wouldn't know either, but she'd make me feel better about not knowing. At least I wasn't the only one making stuff up as I went along.

It was time to go in. I gathered my various flavours of baby porridge into a carrier bag and trudged towards the door.

The woman in front of me was frowning intently at a stack of papers. There were so many that she couldn't hold them all at once and had to rest them on her lap as she thumbed through. I watched in silence as she flipped back and forth between pages of typed and handwritten text. Some were evidently clinic letters, others jotted down during appointments. She narrowed her eyes, as if struggling to decipher something, and made little quiet tutting noises.

She had explained that she was tasked with diagnosing me with borderline personality disorder so that I could join the waiting list to begin the assessment to be approved for the three-month pre-commitment phase before the dialectical behaviour therapy programme, which was followed by a six-month wait, after which I might then be considered a suitable candidate for psychotherapy. The only way to access the therapy was to be diagnosed with BPD by a psychiatrist at the community mental health service. Then I'd be eligible to board the conveyor belt for the assessment and pre-commitment phase, et cetera, et cetera. It all seemed rather protracted and silly, but I knew better than to say so.

She had 'called up' my psychiatric medical notes. I didn't know what that entailed but I imagined her summoning them in some sort of ritual, perhaps around a cauldron, like calling up the spirits of the dead. These notes would help her to decide whether I had BPD. There was also the secondary question of whether I had BPD instead of bipolar or as well as bipolar. We were meeting so that she could deliver the verdict. Then, hopefully, she would make the referral.

So far, it wasn't going well. She couldn't find most of the

notes, and those she could find were muddled and confusing. I wasn't surprised. I didn't envy her this task of interpreting my fifteen years of patienthood. I lived through those years, and I didn't have an interpretation either. These experiences of madness were so bewildering and so fragmented, and the responses to them so various and so fragmented, and all the doctors and services and appointments and treatments were so fragmented, they had fragmented me as a person. None of it made sense.

'But still,' she said, her voice chiming a note of optimism that was transparently false. 'I do have Dr Freyman's notes here, and Dr Radcliffe's. That's something to work with. I'm trying to get a sense of how rapid your mood changes have been over time. That's the key difference. If you have more than a few episodes of mania or depression a year, we'd call that rapid cycling bipolar disorder, but if your mood is changing more frequently than every few weeks, that indicates BPD. So, I've been trying to track your moods over the period between 2007 and 2012, because that's when I have the most information. But it's not very clear at all. It's all a bit patchy, really ...'

She trailed off, muttering as she read, and then picked up again: 'Of course, this is also complicated by the fact that you could have bipolar disorder *and* BPD at the same time – comorbid, we call it.'

It did sound quite morbid. I studied her as the minutes ticked by. She had olive skin, dark hair gathered into a loose bun, and faded brown lipstick. She was, I guessed, about ten years older than me. I wondered if she had grown up nearby. Did she have brothers or sisters? A partner? Kids? What were the chances – in all the vast expanse of the globe and all human history – that she and I should meet in this room, like this? What if we had collided somewhere else? If she were the older sister of a schoolfriend, or if we had studied together at university? What if we'd hiked around Europe together?

Would you like me if you knew me? I asked her in my head. Would I like you? What if you hadn't been tasked with deciding my fate like this? You look as if you would prefer that. I would too. Your coffee is getting cold, by the way.

She sighed. 'I'm not really getting anywhere with this. What's your sense of how often your moods change?'

I had little to say that was useful to her. I supposed there were big moods and little moods, and little moods within the big moods, and what I remember describing to the first counsellor I was sent to in 2001 as 'sharp stabs' of psychological pain. I supposed that a week or a month could have an overall theme of being high or low but there was some variation within that. Essentially, I had no idea, and so I blathered for a while without really knowing what I said. I wanted very much to go back outside, and as I was talking, I thought of grass and sunlight and Arthur laughing in his highchair at the kitchen table. I thought of him until I almost felt rods of light bursting through my fingertips.

The psychiatrist released me with a new diagnosis of BPD and a promise that she would refer me to the personality disorder service. This was progress. She couldn't decide whether I was also bipolar, concluding that the safest option was to 'leave the bipolar where it is' – meaning that I officially had both borderline personality disorder and bipolar disorder.

Bipolar was never mentioned again.

—

Arthur spat out his baby porridge in disgust. As the grey gunk dripped down his chin, I had to admit I didn't blame him. A few weeks later, I tried him on Weetabix. That boy loved Weetabix. He vibrated with excitement whenever he saw me reach into the cereal cupboard. Weetabix dried like cement on the kitchen floor.

Waiting for the personality disorder service appointment letter to arrive, I kept busy. I was still involved in online perinatal peer support, holding virtual hands with the friends in my phone while pinned beneath a sleeping baby. I led Twitter chats, wrote blog posts . . . I was beginning to realise that I had Things to Say, and that I needed to say them, even if I wasn't quite sure what they were yet.

Meanwhile, Hayley and I were having a grand maternity leave, charging around town with our prams. Her start to motherhood had been as fraught as my own: six long weeks of agony trying to breastfeed until she and her son were too ill to continue. Both were healthier and happier after switching to formula, but she was plagued by the same guilt about it that had so troubled me. It was baby formula, for god's sake. A formula specially designed for babies. It wasn't liquid crack. Why were we made to feel that we had failed? Why could I tell Hayley that it was fine, better than fine, that she did a tremendous job under impossible circumstances, and yet I couldn't believe that of myself?

I watched her son dribble more milk over his clothes than went into his mouth and suggested we go and see Sarah at Nature's Mothers. We went together and learned that the issue was another whopping great tongue-tie. One snip and no more dribbling. But Hayley had lost her chance to breastfeed, and she'd lost those early weeks to a blur of pain and misery, just as I had.

'What's that?' I asked her one day in Caffè Nero, one hand cupped around my flat white and the other pointing to an odd-looking package stuffed among the nappies and wipes in her changing bag.

'That's half a Ginsters pasty. I had the other half for breakfast.'

'Ooh, guess what I had for breakfast?'

'What?'

'Meringue.'

With Hayley, I didn't have to pretend to have my shit together. We went to TK Maxx and she tried on some trousers. 'Do I look like MC Hammer?' she hollered across the shop floor. I turned around. She did indeed look like MC Hammer, astonishingly so for a ginger-haired white woman. I tried on the trousers after her, just for a laugh. Then we went to Specsavers and tried glasses on the babies.

Sometimes we went to mother and baby groups at the children's centre, where Hayley held court and I held back and marvelled at her. I still found maternal chit-chat difficult. It was all comparing birth experiences – I'd scurry across the room to be as far away as possible from that conversation unfolding – or it was teething, which is objectively very boring, and how much sleep they'd had or hadn't had. All these women seemed to want to talk about was babies.

Ironically, most of them looked like they'd never had babies. They had the toned stomachs of a nineties girl band, while I practically needed a wheelbarrow for mine. It hung like an apron over my scar, which I couldn't look at, let alone touch. One of the mums from our antenatal class had a C-section the same week I did, and she had just run her first postnatal half-marathon. I still had to turn sideways to sit up in bed. It was all a bit depressing, and I'd rather have had Hayley to myself, but at the same time watching her flinging kindness around like confetti did make me want to cheer.

I was enjoying Arthur more and more each day, although motherhood itself was tiring and expensive and steeped in bullshit. For example, I bought him the 'must-have' teething aid for *fifteen* pounds, only to find that it was a squeaky rubber dog toy. The dog toy for babies was redeemed by his gleeful cackling as I waved it around and sang a special sweary song. In my sleep-starved state, I became the John Lennon of teething accessories. Another original composition was called 'A Great Big Burp (The Trapped Wind Song)'. I'd catch myself singing it even when Arthur wasn't in the room.

I'm horrible at singing, but he was visibly delighted every time I opened my mouth. He looked at me like I was magic, like I was the whole world. In response, every song I've ever known poured out of me, overlapping streams of nursery rhymes, lullabies, hymns, adverts . . . I served up all the background music of existence and he drank it in, wide-eyed. Tunes from my own childhood drifted across the years, one after another, and kept coming. I knew nothing about them until Arthur's expectant little face reconnected some long-disused neural pathway and a song would suddenly spring back to me, complete and fully alive.

When he cut his first tooth, I dutifully brushed that white speck morning and evening, and I sang an old song about a toothbrush to divert him. In the song, a pink toothbrush is the object of the most ardent affections of a blue toothbrush. The blue toothbrush wants to marry the pink toothbrush, who seems to be hesitating, perhaps because toothbrushes don't usually get married. Anyway, that song was originally performed by Max Bygraves, a man I had not thought about in a long time. Nan had a VHS tape of his *Sing-a-long-a War Years*, starring an elderly Max in an ARP Home Front helmet.

Other favourites I'd learned at two or three years old while buttoned inside Nan's cardigan. I felt again how mohair tingled against my cheek when I first encountered cheery classics like 'Molly Malone' and 'Oh My Darling, Clementine'. Hardly suitable nursery staples: everyone was dead or about to be. The deliciously spooky 'The Old Woman Stood at the Churchyard Gate' recounted a dialogue between a woman and three corpses and ended in a loud scream. Arthur, buttoned into my cardigan, was enthralled, and it was as if Nan were there. We were cocooned together: the ghost of my toddler-self and the ghost of her voice in mine, an echo. I was held between Nan and Arthur, who would never meet and were meeting there, in me.

It began to dawn on me that much of my nondescript anguish had been simply the bitter ache of missing her. After she died, the thoughts I would have spoken to her went unspoken, and then I stopped having them altogether. Perhaps it was less painful that way, or perhaps it was just that there was nowhere for them to go. A channel blocked, and I lost access to some essential part of myself. I don't think I had really grieved. I don't think I knew how. There was just an absence, a void that took on its own shape and overshadowed everything.

I thought about Nan, and I missed her, straightforwardly.

four

One day I was in a charity shop, and they had an enormous china dog, about the size of a real Staffie. I wanted to buy it for her collection and present it to her. It would have been so funny. I left it in the shop and walked home, thinking, If only I could get to her.

As soon as someone dies, they're stationary while you're steadily moving forward in time, whether you want to or not. They get further and further away. I can't remember the sound of Nan's voice. I know that if I heard it, I would recognise it immediately, but I can't hear it in my head any more. I hate that. I hate that every day the world contains fewer things that she knew, and more that she didn't. Arthur, for one.

Something in me that had frozen when Nan died was beginning to thaw, but I hadn't noticed, not yet. My hopes were still pinned firmly to DBT and the personality disorder service. Swaying from side to side and watching the flutter of Arthur's sleepy eyelids, I sang to him the third verse of 'Amazing Grace'.

Through many dangers, toils, and snares
we have already come,
but grace has brought us safe thus far
and grace will lead us home.

Pernicious Motivations

It is well known that a large group of patients fit frankly nei-
ther into the psychotic nor into the psychoneurotic group, and
that this border line group of patients is extremely difficult to
handle effectively by any psychotherapeutic method.
> Adolph Stern (1938), 'Psychoanalytic
> Investigation of and Therapy in the Border Line
> Group of Neuroses', *The Psychoanalytic Quarterly*[1]

In retrospect, it is notable how the failures of psychoanalytic
psychotherapies were explained solely by the borderline patient's
pernicious motivations.
> John G. Gunderson (2009), 'Borderline
> Personality Disorder: Ontogeny of a Diagnosis',
> *American Journal of Psychiatry*[2]

Late summer 2014

I don't know that it was grace that led me to the personality disorder service, but I got the letter and turned up
for my first assessment. The service was housed downstairs
in the hospital building where I'd been incarcerated less

than two years before. I should have heeded the bunting of red flags fluttering along the length and breadth of this entire process. In hindsight, it's a bit like when people in scary films go to an abandoned mansion on an ancient burial ground or stay in a derelict hotel in the middle of nowhere. The building is silhouetted against a dark sky, and as they approach, we hear the ominous opening chords of Beethoven's Fifth.

I was defiantly hopeful, even as I held my breath stepping into the building in case it still smelt of that heady combination of bleach and human misery. The therapists here were going to be the experts I'd been looking for all my life. They understood people like me, and they knew how to help. I was willing to work hard. This was how it would be done. It had to be, because otherwise I was out of ideas.

The waiting room of this last-chance saloon was dominated by a large, unframed painting. It depicted — and I shit you not here — a Victorian child dressed as a clown.* There he was, posed awkwardly against a chair, in his blue-and-yellow harlequin bodysuit with a ruff around his neck. His expression was blank, stark, as if he'd recently witnessed unspeakable acts of violence. His feet and the fringed bottom half of the chair were sketched but not coloured in.

I have an unusually high tolerance for creepy things. I've learned to be careful about sharing photos of my doll collection, for example, because people get spooked, or

---

* Since I wrote this, the painting in question has been identified as an amateur copy of Picasso's *Paul in a Clown Suit* from the 1920s, so Paul is not Victorian but he is still quite creepy.

they make jokes about dolls sneaking around malevolently in the middle of the night. One of my dolls is actually a clown; his name is Ambrose Snelgrove. He has a wind-up music box embedded in his chest and it does occasionally let out the odd nocturnal jangle. That doesn't bother me in the slightest, but I freely admit that this painting freaked me out. It was the boy's face, white with shock.

I snapped a photo on my phone and sent it to Jon. I thought of him as he had been when I left, on the sofa with Arthur on his lap. I thought of the dishes in the sink, and the playmat strewn with toys. I wanted to go home. I could go home. No one would stop me if I walked out.

The clown boy whispered horrors through pursed lips as I considered my options. I tried to think calmly, but I couldn't ignore him, flicking his eyes upward, rolling them back, gesturing with one tiny finger to the glittering floors above my head. I remembered the woman who had slept three beds down from me in the dormitory, how she got up one night and started slinging CDs like frisbees out of the window. She had incredible aim: those windows only opened half an inch. The CDs shone on the gravel and on the branches of the nearest tree, like Christmas decorations. She stood at the window, hooting and cheering, until they grabbed her and pinned her to the floor, and a nurse snarled at me to get back into bed.

That was not going to be me in thirty years. I was not going to bounce like a demented pinball in and out of the bin for the rest of my life while Arthur missed me and got sadder and stranger and more fucked-up. I just wasn't going to allow that to happen. Here was an opportunity, and it might not be ideal, but I was going to seize that opportunity and make the best of it. I was going to show up week after bloody week, do the work, identify and fix whatever my problems were, and be Arthur's mum. Whole galleries of weird paintings could line up and give me the side-eye and point at bad memories all day long, and it wasn't going to make the slightest difference. I was staying put.

Soon I followed a woman with impossibly high heels through a labyrinth of corridors. *Clippity clippity clop*, she went, echoing. I marvelled at how she walked, so quickly and deftly, as I plodded behind in my Doc Martens. I imagined myself in shoes like hers, saw myself swaying with arms out for balance like a child walking along a wall. I heard the splintering crack of my chin as it hit the floor. Ouch. In reality, I wouldn't even have got the shoes on. My feet are rectangular – 'brick feet', my brother once memorably called them – and my toes splay out as they bear my weight. I should like to be an elegant, giraffe-like woman in beautiful shoes but even my imagination won't take me that far.

We reached our allocated room, set up in the usual way – chairs, small table, box of tissues, tired-looking plant. I was outnumbered two to one: to my right was another therapist, perched on the edge of her seat with a clipboard and biro. I said hello but I couldn't take my eyes off the woman who had led me in. It wasn't just the five-inch stilettos, but her glossy black hair scraped back and piled above her head, the precision of her eyeliner, her lipliner, her nails … Everything about her swept smoothly to a sharp point. She reminded me of a ballet teacher I had when I was little, her long fingernails the colour of a fire engine. If you were stood in the wrong place, as I usually was, she would take hold of your forearm and lead you across the room. I felt the pressure of the tips of her nails on my chubby little wrists. It hurt but it never quite punctured the skin.

Rubbing my arm, I tuned back into the personality disorder therapists, who were showing me their paperwork. There was a series of columns in a table which stretched over pages and pages. On the far left was a list of criteria, while the other columns were space for notes about the extent to which each item applied to me. This was to confirm the diagnosis and my suitability for treatment. I had seen these criteria before, of course. I'd looked them up online and pored over them more times than I cared to recount. The introductory paragraph read as follows:

Personality disorder characterised by a definite tendency to act impulsively and without consideration of the consequences; the mood is unpredictable and capricious. There is a liability to outbursts of emotion and an incapacity to control the behavioural explosions. There is a tendency to quarrelsome behaviour and to conflicts with others, especially when impulsive acts are thwarted or censored. Two types may be distinguished: the impulsive type, characterised predominantly by emotional instability and lack of impulse control, and the borderline type, characterised in addition by disturbances in self-image, aims, and internal preferences, by chronic feelings of emptiness, by intense and unstable interpersonal relationships, and by a tendency to self-destructive behaviour, including suicide gestures and attempts.[3]

In the table below were nine criteria:

1. *Frantic efforts to avoid real or imagined abandonment. Note: Do not include suicidal or self-mutilating behaviour covered in Criterion 5.*

2. *A pattern of unstable and intense interpersonal relationships characterised by alternating between extremes of idealisation and devaluation.*

3. *Identity disturbance: markedly and persistently unstable self-image or sense of self.*

4. *Impulsivity in at least two areas that are potentially self-damaging (e.g., spending, sex, substance abuse, reckless driving, binge eating). Note: Do not include suicidal or self-mutilating behaviour covered in Criterion 5.*

5. *Recurrent suicidal behaviour, gestures, or threats, or self-mutilating behaviour.*

6. *Affective instability due to a marked reactivity of mood (e.g., intense episodic dysphoria, irritability, or anxiety usually lasting a few hours and only rarely more than a few days).*

7. *Chronic feelings of emptiness.*

8. *Inappropriate, intense anger or difficulty controlling anger (e.g., frequent displays of temper, constant anger, recurrent physical fights).*

9. *Transient, stress-related paranoid ideation or severe dissociative symptoms.*[4]

We had two appointments to get through these, and I needed to tick five out of nine boxes to qualify for treatment. And so off we went, tick tick tick.

When nudged to muse about my friendships, I didn't focus on Harriet or Nick or anyone else who has been a consistent loving presence since my teens, but on anyone who had distanced themselves or disappeared. I described everyone who had ever said I was horrible, and the friendships that had started well but then, seemingly inexplicably, gone south. That was clearly what I was supposed to talk about and so that was what I talked about, because even after all this time, I just wanted to be a good girl and do as I was told so that I would get better.

And I could do this. It was easy to dredge up ancient history and claim total responsibility. It was all too easy to hypothesise that I am horrid even when I don't mean to be, that I am deep down, intrinsically bad, and that my good intentions count for naught. That was always my greatest fear, and for the first time I said it out loud. The two women nodded. They wrote it down.

'And what's your sexual orientation?' asked the one who had led me into the room. Evidently, she was asking the questions.

'I'm, er, bisexual.'

She looked up briefly, raising one perfect eyebrow. 'Oh, really?'

'Yeah.'

'But you said you have a son. Is that correct?'

'That's right.'

'And you're married?'

'Yes.'

'To a man?'

'Yes.'

'Your son's father?'

'Yes.'

'So, you seem to be confused there ... around your sexual identity. Would you say that's the case?'

'Not really, no.'

I tried to keep the annoyance out of my voice, but I could see she had spotted it. I held her gaze. Her eyes were ice-blue and thickly lined in pencil.

'There's no need to be aggressive,' she said softly.

'I'm not. Sorry. I just mean – it's not like I'm indecisive

about whether I'm gay or not. That's not what bisexual means – not that I'm trying to tell you – of course you know what it means. I'm just bi. Always have been.'

Her eyes widened as if I'd said something outrageous. Did she think I'd been some sort of randy toddler? We were less than twenty minutes in.

'Since my teens, anyway. I mean, that was when I first worked it out and I've just been so ever since. It doesn't change – whether I'm in a relationship with a woman or a man, I'm still the same, but people tend to assume that, like, if I'm with a woman I must be gay, and if with a man I must be straight, but that doesn't actually make it so, and what they assume doesn't really matter – at least not to me . . . It's not really anyone's business.'

'Uh huh,' she said slowly. 'You're describing quite a range of sexual partners there. Would you say that you're promiscuous?'

'The chance would be a fine thing,' I quipped in panic.

Nobody smiled. They didn't even look up. They were both writing now, faster and faster. I realised with mounting horror that not only had my joke fallen flat, but they were probably writing something like '*would be promiscuous only nobody wants to shag her*'.

I hurriedly injected, 'I mean, of course not, no. As you mentioned, I'm married. I've been married for five years.'

I thought my marriedness would be sufficient to shield me from further discussion of this nature, but she pressed on.

'And are you having extramarital affairs?'

'God, no.'

My Friday night was not what she thought it was. It was me reading Terry Pratchett in a shawl more often than not.

What did she think I did with Arthur when I was out on the town?

'And what about before you were married?'

'It would have been difficult to have extramarital affairs before I was married.'

She put down her pen and I heard it land gently on the paper.

Oh, big mistake. Big, big mistake. This was just the sort of smart-arsery that got me into trouble at Maplewood.

There was a long pause.

I'd blown it, clearly. No therapy for me. Fucking hell, why did I ruin everything? Why did I torch every chance I was offered?

Eventually, she took a slow, deep breath.

'Would you like to continue this assessment?'

'Yes, please,' I replied in a small voice.

'You may be used to being argumentative and disruptive, Laura, but we don't stand for that here. If you want our help, you're going to have to control yourself.'

'Look, I'm not trying – Sorry. I just – I feel a bit like I'm on trial here …'

The woman seated to my right deftly flipped forward a few pages. I could just make out that she had swapped to the section for 'inappropriate, intense anger'. She had tiny, cramped handwriting.

'Do you now?' There was that soft voice again. 'Perhaps you'd like to tell us a bit more about that.'

'No, no, it's fine. Sorry. I just meant – this is quite difficult. Sorry.'

'Right. I'll try again. Would you say that your sexual behaviour has been promiscuous in the past?'

My voice caught in my throat. 'I – I dunno. I mean,

when I was a student, there were some . . . It depends on what you count as promiscuous.'

If I cringed hard enough, would I turn inside out? My hands hung uselessly in my lap, two tangled gardens of nerve and sinew.

'I see you're determined to be evasive here. It's understandable to feel shame about these sorts of activities. Perhaps we can come back to this later. Let's move on for now, shall we? Have you ever taken any illegal drugs?'

'Um, I've smoked cannabis a few times, years ago. It was being passed around. And, uh, I did try ecstasy once at a party.'

'Only once?'

'Yeah, it was rubbish. I drank a lot of Ribena and watched a DVD without being able to follow it. It was some comedy series. I can't remember what. And there was a guy there who kept arguing with himself in the mirror. Nobody seemed to be having much fun. So I didn't try it again.'

More furious note-taking.

'And have you ever shoplifted?'

'Ugh, again, once. I was about fifteen and out with my friend Harriet. We met up in Winchester, I think, and ended up stealing some novelty plasters from Claire's Accessories. I felt so guilty that a week later I went back – to another branch of Claire's nearer home, in an entirely different city – and I left £1.50 on the shelf by the plasters. I was convinced I was going to be arrested on the spot.'

They looked so serious I half thought they were going to arrest me. Better not mention the delicious little coconut mushrooms I used to snaffle out of Woolworth's Pick 'n' Mix in the nineties, or they'd march me to a police station right there and then. 'Thank god, you've caught Pick 'n' Mix Kid!' a policeman would exclaim. 'We've been after her for twenty years! The reward is yours. Come this way. Steve, call the detective constable.'

It was dawning on me that this was a foregone conclusion. Whatever I said – or didn't – could be mapped onto the nine criteria. They were a bit like a horoscope: constructed to be universally relatable, just enough of a reflective surface that anyone could see themselves if they looked hard.* But really this was a *good* thing, because it meant I could have the therapy. And, yes, this questioning was unpleasant and sort of farcical, really, but I just had to get through it and not do anything daft like storming out of there, and then I could have that specialist support.

Therapy wouldn't be easy, I knew that, and this was good practice. A chance to show that I'm someone who can stick it out, who is willing to face up to the unlikable parts of themselves. One day I would write a book called *How DBT Changed My Life* and people would read it who felt desperate and unreachable, just like me. DBT was the lighthouse to guide us all home.

——

At the second session, the chief inquisitor arrived on crutches. I asked her what happened, and she replied, 'I

---

* The horoscope analogy is perfect but is not my own: researcher Rachel Rowan Olive included it in the materials for her one-day training course: 'I is for Insult: Questioning Borderline Personality Disorder'. That's also where I came across the two papers quoted in the epigraph. Rachel's work has been instrumental in helping me and so many others to make sense of our encounters with personality disorder. See www.rachelrowanolive.com

have a broken foot.' I made what I hoped was a sympathetic noise.

I had spent a long time analysing what made the first session such a car crash. I decided I must not have explained myself very well. I gave them the wrong idea about me, which was why they clearly thought I was an absolute wrong 'un and why it all felt so squirmy and gross. With time to think and prepare, I would do better.

My theory was that the criteria we were covering – impulsivity, self-harm, suicidality, mood swings – had a common root cause in my case. That cause was pain: mental and emotional pain. It's not like you can take ibuprofen for that sort of pain, and yet, like physical pain, when it becomes intolerable, it does affect your judgement. Making it stop, or making it hurt less, becomes such a priority that you'll do almost anything. The inventor of dialectical behaviour therapy, Marsha Linehan, wrote that people with BPD are like burns victims: without emotional skin, they feel agony at the slightest touch or movement. That was exactly what it was like. I was so bloody sensitive, always had been.

'You've certainly done your homework,' mused the one with the broken foot. She didn't say that like it was a good thing. 'We're not here to listen to you make excuses for yourself. The aim of these sessions is to confirm the diagnosis and decide if you're a good candidate for the therapy programme. Let's stick to going through these criteria.'

'Suicidal behaviour' was an obvious tick. I was asked to number how many times I had tried to end my life, and I couldn't. I wasn't sure. Another tick for 'self-mutilating behaviour': I had been hurting myself in various ways since I was eleven or twelve. As much as I felt that many of these criteria were applicable to everyone to some extent, I couldn't deny that they might as well have put my name down as criterion five.

I was still valiantly and stupidly trying to explain myself as we went along. While conceding that, yes, of course I wanted to stop self-harming because obviously it's horrible, hurting yourself on purpose, I had to point out that I wanted to stop because I no longer needed it rather than because other people thought I should stop. Other people were so rarely aware of what I was doing anyway. I had enough basic knowledge of anatomy to make sure I didn't fuck myself up too badly. I'd been self-harming for so long, and it was such an integral part of how I dealt with the world, that I couldn't really imagine a version of myself who never did that.

'You should know,' she replied, 'that if you are accepted onto the programme, you'll sign a contract waiving your right to hurt yourself in any way.'

'Wow.'

'Remember that we have a lot of experience in dealing with people with personality disorders. We know that they can be very manipulative in getting their own way, and in finding reasons why the rules don't apply to them. We enforce our contracts absolutely and without exception.'

The contract, she explained, had various clauses listing not only what I could and couldn't do, both during and outside of therapy, but also any topics I was not permitted to discuss. There were unspecified 'consequences' for breaking this contract. The ultimate consequence was withdrawal of therapy and all support.

I held my tongue – literally held it between my teeth. It felt like I'd burned it on pizza.

The more likely it seemed that I would be accepted onto the therapy programme, the more mental gymnastics were required to assure myself that I wanted to be there. I thought of the supposedly banana-flavoured antibiotic medicine I used to hide from behind the sofa when I was a child. Even the sight of the bottle made me heave, its luminous tinge. But from the high vantage point of adulthood, I could be glad that my parents forced me to swallow it so that I recovered from my tonsillitis and lived to hide another day. Now I was the parent. I had been asking for this medicine for so long. I wasn't going to bolt because I didn't like the taste.

I nodded along as they outlined the three-month precommitment phase, followed by fourteen months of one-to-one therapy one morning and one afternoon each week, plus group sessions, daily journaling, and constant practice and application of the DBT skills. All this was to 'stabilise' me – like putting jelly in the fridge, I supposed – and then I would be left to 'settle' for six months, after which I'd be considered robust enough to start psychotherapy.

I held myself still and steady, my lower back anchored into the seat.

We were approaching the last of the nine criteria. 'Would you say that you're prone to temper tantrums?' she asked.

'I don't – I don't think so. I mean, I do get angry, but I'm more likely to take it out on myself.'

Predictably, the note-taker flipped back several pages.

'You wouldn't say that you ever have outbursts, as such? Perhaps raise your voice or say cruel things?'

'Well, not never. Admittedly I did get into some right strops as a teenager.'

I could hear the rustling of paper to my right again.

'Hmm. In fact, we've witnessed some of your "strops" already, don't you think?'

What I thought was that I'd quite like to go back to being bipolar.

'Let me ask you something else,' she continued. 'Do you think that you're cleverer than other people?'

I hesitated. That wasn't on the list.

'Well, some other people, surely. I'm not the cleverest person in the world but statistically . . . I mean, I'd hazard a guess I'm in the top half? Cleverness is such a multi-faceted thing, anyway. But, yeah, admittedly there have been times when I was talking to people – often mental health professionals, actually – and I was conscious that . . .'

Realising too late that this was an extraordinarily stupid answer, I let my voice drop.

'Conscious of what, Laura?'

'Well, that they weren't very bright. But I don't mean . . . Christ, do you have a shovel?'

I looked to each of them in turn, as if in appeal. The note-taker didn't so much as glance up. Her colleague's face was set, her mouth a hard line beneath its lipstick.

Eventually she said, 'I'm not sure we should have you in a group-therapy setting, Laura.'

'Why not?'

'I think you might be unkind to the other members of the group.'

'I – I don't think I would do that.'

'You might not mean to, I suppose, but that wouldn't make any difference to the people harmed by you.'

I was starting to hate her – both of them, in fact – and this, too, was evidence of the conclusion to which all roads had been leading, not only during the assessment, but throughout my whole life. I had a disordered personality, that much was obvious. More than that, I was so toxic that I couldn't be trusted to interact with other human beings at all. I would effectively have to be quarantined for the duration of my treatment. I hadn't given them the wrong idea about me. They were simply able to see past my own self-delusion.

'Would you be able to help me still, if I didn't come to the group?'

'No,' she said firmly. 'The group is part of the programme.'

'Perhaps I could just sit quietly and not say anything? And then I could still learn from the group but without . . . being a danger?'

'I think that would be best, to begin with. We can review it with your therapist as you go.'

I kept thinking of little Arthur at home, his soft blond wisps of angel hair, his skin so fair and soft that something hardened broke in me every time I touched him. I thought of his sudden laughter and the way he sprawled out when he napped, with his beloved Chewy Bear in his mouth. What had I brought him into?

The next day, while Arthur was sleeping, I searched on Amazon for books about parenting with BPD. Ideally, I was looking for a book entitled *How Not to Fuck Up Your Child's Life When You Are the Absolute Worst*.

I didn't find any advice, or reassurance. I did find the following titles:

Borderline Personality: My Torment from a Toxic BPD Mother (subtitle: *A Shattered Childhood*)
Borderline Personality Disorder: Growing Up with a BPD Mother or Dad – Our Childhood from Hell
Surviving a Borderline Parent: How to Heal Your Childhood Wounds and Build Trust, Boundaries, and Self-Esteem

Perhaps I needed to turn to something more authoritative. Next, I came across a report by the Royal College of Psychiatrists, *Parents as patients: supporting the needs of patients who are parents and their children.*

A substantial proportion of self-reported child abusers are diagnosed with personality disorder and it is a diagnosis commonly made by professionals reporting in child protection proceedings . . . In one small study of maltreating mothers, half of the sample had a diagnosis of a personality disorder . . . Parents who have a personality disorder are likely to struggle for three reasons:

1 having a child will stimulate their attachment system,
2 their capacity to manage and self-soothe their own arousal is limited, and
3 they will not be able to soothe their own child's distress, but instead respond with hostility or fear.

This then leads to a vicious cycle, in which the child gets more distressed, and the parent becomes either more frightened or frightening; which in turn makes it likely that the child will become insecurely attached … The presence of personality disorder therefore compromises parenting to the same extent as severe mental illness does, and perhaps even more.[5]

'*I'm so sorry,*' I whispered, sitting on the carpet with one hand through the bars of the cot. '*I love you.*'

Arthur breathed gently, one hand curled around my index finger. I could almost hear his mind whirring, becoming.

I love you. I'm sorry. Even that sounded manipulative. I could hear it – the mind-twisting cruelty of anything and everything that came out of my mouth. I jammed my other fist between my teeth and bit down hard.

That Time May Find Its Sound Again

Burn, glare, old sun, so long unseen,
That time may find its sound again, and cleanse
Whatever it is that a wound remembers
After the healing ends.

Weldon Kees, 'Small Prayer'[1]

Winter 2014–15

Rubber-stamped for therapy, I had been on a waiting list around four months when a letter landed on the doormat, jumbled up with my Christmas cards. I was to come to a meeting with 'the head of services' on 30 December. There was no further explanation. I had an uneasy suspicion that the purpose of this meeting might be to continue the discussion about my suitability for group therapy and any risk I posed to other patients. Perhaps the issue had been escalated.

The temptation to consign the letter and its contents to the recycling bin was a powerful one, but I remained determined to face my dragons so that Arthur didn't have to. If, to confront my internal dragons, I must first face an external dragon – and I sensed that this head of services would not be a cuddly individual – well, then, bring it on. I wrote and wrote in my various notebooks to gear myself up, urging courage.

Those diaries are a mixture of notes penned at an awkward angle from beneath a dozing child, and more fluent, inky introspection from when I stayed up very late, despite being desert-eyed and a little wild with tiredness, just for the quiet and the solitude. I craved aloneness, although I was lonely. Hayley had gone back to work. The late, great, drunkenly glowing nights at the pub were a thing of the past, and the regulars moving on, one by one. I spent my evenings lamenting to my notebooks about a relentless stream of nappies, bottles, washing up, laundry, meals, emails . . . I seemed to be constantly descaling the kettle.

Arthur was cutting teeth and dealt with it by honking like an angry goose. I felt for him because he was little and in pain, but also the noise made me want to rip my skin off. I prayed to every god I could think of that he'd sleep through the night, knowing full well that he wouldn't sleep through the night. Arthur was still a beacon, my golden boy, and there were bright moments – but mostly it was grey, grey, dragging days, endless nights, and a nameless longing.

My fieldnotes of motherhood were interspersed with hand-wringing about the implications of a personality disorder diagnosis: that I – '*a toxic, draining, destructive presence*' – was in closest proximity to the people I loved most. '*How will I damage Arthur, how will I further damage Jon, as the years pass? I am all good intentions but poison anyone who gets close.*'

I carried on like this, at least in part, because the

personality disorder assessment had confirmed my original hypothesis that I was to blame for everything that had happened. Where I couldn't see that I had directly caused it, I must have indirectly caused it. I attracted it. I deserved it. If bad things happened to me, that was because I was bad news.

I could never regret having Arthur, but I so regretted that he had me. My only hope – *his* only hope of having a mother who was not inherently abusive – was the DBT programme, and so I was resolute that they would take me even though I felt sick every time I thought of going back. Somehow, I would find the resources within myself to stay the course. Therapy twice a week, plus group sessions, phone calls, constant skills practice . . . It sounded exhausting, and I was already exhausted, but it was the only route I could see. If I could envision it, if I could describe this process and the wise, sober, unflappable person who would replace me at the end of it, maybe I could summon her into being. Maybe Arthur wouldn't have to remember this incarnation of me at all.

His first Christmas dawned. I carried him up to the attic bedroom and presented him with his stocking. He was captivated, instead, by the box of tissues on my bedside table. He pulled the tissues out one by one, delighted with each. They did make a lovely whooshing noise as they came out of the box. We waved tissues around for a while, and I briefly forgot that it was five days and counting until I had to go back to the personality disorder service. That was a strange, slow Christmas – family visiting and Arthur in his little red jumper and nervous dread soaking into everything like booze-drenched fruitcake.

When I went to the meeting with the head of services,

it turned out to be my launch into the three-month 'pre-commitment phase' of DBT. The big kahuna was my therapist. Bizarrely, I remember nothing about that meeting. In my notebook, I wrote that the therapist's name was Angela, and that she'd banished any lingering doubts about the diagnosis: '*I describe things about myself that I have always considered to be odd or unique, and she nods away and says it's all very typical.*' Aside from this, I couldn't tell you anything about Angela, what she said to me or what we did together. My diaries skimmed over our sessions, and all I can recall from several months of weekly appointments is one time when we were side-tracked into an interesting discussion about regional dialects.

I don't know why I didn't write about DBT at a time when I was recording almost everything that flitted between my ears. I don't know why I don't remember it. I suspect this amnesia may have something to do with an unfortunate defensive habit in which part of my brain would go offline as soon as I was sequestered into these strangely intimate one-to-ones with anyone wearing an NHS lanyard. And yet I can recall that original assessment in all its stinging, squirming detail. Perhaps that was what did it. Or perhaps it was that Arthur's first birthday was on the horizon.

———

Birthdays after birth trauma are strange. They're a celebration of a much-loved child, and they're also 'crappiversaries' – a concise if rather twee name for the anniversary of a traumatic event. However fiercely you ignore a crappiversary, it always finds a way to announce itself. The body rides the seasons like a carousel. It remembers, and it knows.

I had been in pain, in and around the incision across my pelvis, for almost a full year. Before Arthur's birth, pain was something short-lived: a twisted ankle, a stubbed toe, a headache, an ear infection. This was a different pain that was background noise, like someone drilling the street outside the front door. It was a sharp, hairy prickling at the edges of my scar, and a pulling sensation, as if my ovaries were hooked onto elastic. I still rolled onto my side to get out of bed in the morning. There were chairs I could not get out of gracefully. I was used to it. In a sense, I was astonished to be up and about and moving through the world almost as I had before, astonished at my body's ability to piece itself back together.

After prescriptions for painkillers and two inconclusive ultrasounds of my uterus, a GP offered to refer me to a pain clinic. A pain clinic – a clinic of pain – did not sound good at all. Like a torture institution. My understanding was that a pain clinic was where they taught you to put up with it. I didn't need to be taught to put up with it. I *was* putting up with it. I was the queen of putting up with it, and of getting on with it. I could probably have taught them a thing or two. It became more wearing to keep asking than to put up indefinitely. If it couldn't be helped, then that was that, I supposed. But I hoped it wouldn't hurt this way for the rest of my life. The rest of my life was potentially quite a long time.

There were emotional twinges too – soaring ones, bittersweet – at saying goodbye to my baby and hello to my toddler. Every day was a milestone, momentous in its own small way: a new word, the ability to sing snatches of a recognisable tune, the realisation that if he pulled his plastic train backward, it would then scoot forward. I did a wardrobe changeover and found that the clothes in a carrier bag onto which I had sellotaped a Post-it note marked 'HUGE', for the dim and distant future, fit Arthur perfectly. I held them up in astonishment against the clothes which had gone into the wardrobe a few months before.

Arthur's birth was still a heap of muddled memories, a patchwork quilt that wouldn't stitch together, but since we'd left the mother and baby unit, it had kept a safe distance. Most days it felt like it had happened to someone else. When I looked back, it was with some shock – how dark and odd it all was, how little I had understood.

But as the birthday drew closer, I began to feel as if the events of the previous year were still happening somewhere else. I felt like I was being pulled into them. And I felt guilty. Arthur's birthday was Arthur's birthday, not my birth-trauma anniversary. Only a wicked, selfish, personality-disordered mother would make her child's birthday all about herself by fixating on her birth experience. I was *not* going to be that mother.

So I planned a big party. I would fill the house with people. Arthur would have balloons and taste chocolate cake for the first time. This was going to be *fun*, damn it.

'*Narcissist,*' I breathed every time the thought occurred to me that I would rather be doing almost anything other than arranging a party.

The panic that had been gently receding since the mother and baby unit was flooding back. I continued to ignore it and berate myself by turns, like Canute shouting at the sea. Once again, my body became a siren. I would act as if trivial things were emergencies because it made sense, then, that my muscles were tense, and my mouth was parched, and I could hear my heart banging away.

Missed a bus? Emergency! Lost a sock? Emergency! I was ridiculous, and I knew it.

I irritated myself and everyone around me, Jon most of all. The crosser he was, the more frantic I became, and his crossness became the new emergency. Whether I was defensive or tried to placate him or tried to explain – whatever I did, it made him crosser still. Soon he only had to enter the room and I'd start panicking internally. Then I'd panic about failing to conceal the fact that I was panicking. I was so afraid that my body, or my tone of voice, would betray me, and that Jon would snap or sigh or roll his eyes. Which of course he did, often, because he's only human and I was a nightmare to live with.

I could see that this spike in anxiety probably had something to do with birth trauma, and yet I didn't recall feeling anxious or afraid at all during labour, or while Arthur was being born. If anything, it was the opposite. I didn't remember any emotions. It was more like static frames, a series of paintings along a wall.

———

The evening before Arthur's birthday was still and dark. All day the air had been thrumming with spring trying to happen, thick cloud and sunshine competing for the sky. Dusk had long passed, and the blinds on the window behind me shut out the streetlights. There was only the orange glow of the night-light in the corner. I was in the rocking chair facing Arthur's cot. He dozed, sprawled across my lap. His toes twitched inside his cotton sleeping bag.

I was waiting for him to settle into a deeper sleep before I set him down. Any transfer of sleeping baby from warm arms to flat surface was always a risk. He could go from sleeping baby to screaming baby in the seconds that it took me to creep backwards while holding my breath. Best to wait until he was properly out for the count before attempting anything. He was well on the way. Soon I'd be heading downstairs. I was tired, I realised, and a little thirsty. I lay back for a moment and closed my eyes.

The thirst was everything and everything was pain. When I forced my eyes open, it was like looking through a thin film of PVA glue. Faces hovered over me. My lips parted uselessly, and there was Jon with the white disposable cup and the water spilling down my hospital gown and the pink plastic straw and the whole world tumbling and rolling into the distance.

I jerked forwards, and as I did, I saw Arthur – fair-haired, sleeping-bagged, and fast asleep, almost one year old – and I yelled in surprise, nearly throwing him off my lap. Thankfully my wait-it-out bedtime transfer method was so effective that he stirred and moaned only briefly, soothed as soon as I cradled him against my chest. But I needed to wait again. I hunched forwards, clutching him a little too tightly, and I held my eyes open, afraid to blink.

'This is Arthur's bedroom,' I whispered to myself. 'It's Thursday evening.' I told myself the date, and that I was twenty-seven years old, and that Arthur was exactly 364 days old, and that we were here, and that we were safe.

The room was strangely silent. The street outside seemed deserted: no cars passing, no doors slamming, no voices. I thought of the woman screaming outside the window when I was in the birth pool, screaming as if her life depended on it. Except that she wasn't screaming because she didn't exist. There was no woman. Still, I almost expected to hear her again. I listened to the silence.

'That was then, and this is now,' I whispered aloud again, as if to ward her off.

'That was then, and this is now.'

As I came downstairs and into the kitchen, Jon was cooking dinner. He stood with his back to me, stirring a pan on the hob.

'When Arthur was born,' I started.

Jon didn't turn around, but I could feel that he was listening.

'When Arthur was trying to be born, did you bring me a cup of water? With a straw? Because I couldn't drink it otherwise and it had spilled?'

'Uh, yeah, that's right.'

'Oh. I – I just remembered that.'

There was a pause.

'Thanks,' I added. 'Belatedly.'

'Er, you're welcome. Do you want some wine?'

'Yes. I would love some wine. I want some squash too.'

I ran the tap and water sloshed into the bottom of the glass, diluting my blackcurrant squash. I gulped it down without stopping for air and immediately refilled the glass. The squash was cold and sweet and refreshing, and I never wanted to not be able to get myself a drink, not ever again.

Then I went to pick up Arthur's toys, scattered across the floor of the front room. As I lifted a painted wooden caterpillar from the playmat and turned to toss it into the toybox, I noticed that my hand was trembling.

I hosted a party. I sat on the floor with Arthur in my lap as we opened his presents. I ate more than my share of Gruffalo birthday cake. I wiped down the highchair and sang songs and changed nappies as if nothing was wrong. Maybe nothing *was* wrong. It was only that I felt like a bystander, observing myself, that funny woman always so busy with this and with that.

Did I talk to Angela about Arthur's birthday? Did I tell her that I was having flashbacks again? Was there a DBT skill, was there a worksheet for that? I have no idea. It was like there was an alternative version of me who only existed intermittently. She handled the DBT appointments, and she kept her own counsel, releasing me to care for Arthur, to run the home, to write when I could, and to think my own thoughts.

There was a further complicating factor: I didn't know if I could complete the DBT programme after all. The landlord had informed us that our home was going to be sold from under us again. He said something about 'changes in stamp duty' although I had little idea what this meant beyond that it was probably not anything to do with postage stamps. Jon and I couldn't afford to buy the house, not even nearly. If we took ourselves away from Surrey's commuter belt, we stood a better chance of buying somewhere eventually. In the meantime, renting elsewhere, we could afford two bedrooms plus space for Jon to work from home. And we would be less likely to be booted out every five minutes. And it would be good to be near family. Those considerations – combined with a growing restlessness and staleness, a sense that our life as it was had passed its expiration date – made a compelling case for moving back to Southampton.

But that would disrupt and delay my personality disorder treatment. I'd be out of catchment for the service I was under and would have to migrate to a different one. When murmurs first began about stamp duty, I hoped to postpone our move long enough to get those fourteen months of DBT under my belt. Then maybe I could wave them at whatever gatekeeper and go straight into psychotherapy once we were settled in Southampton. Except, of course, that was never going to work. It was far too straightforward. And the landlord wanted us out. I was going to have to speak to Angela.

Mother City

A giving up is a making room.

Laura Varnam, 'A New Woman
at Beowulf's Funeral Pyre'[1]

Summer and autumn 2015

As we retrieved the cardboard boxes from under the stairs and started packing up our lives again, I replayed the final conversation with Angela over in my mind. Once we were settled in Southampton, I was to go to the GP and request a referral for a personality disorder service. Then I would join a waiting list and start the assessment process all over again. It was less like Snakes and Ladders and more like Frustration, if you've ever played that. Suddenly you're bumped not even back to Start, but to a limbo area where you can't progress to Start for an indefinite period of time.

We rented a house in a Victorian terrace along a busy main road, just a couple of streets away from my parents. It was all achingly familiar. As I trod the pavements, they seemed to vibrate with the step of my same feet in jelly shoes, in Clarks T-bar school shoes, in chunky-heeled lace-up Kickers, right up to the purple floral Doc Martens I wore when I left at eighteen. I would have to work out how to be an adult in this place.

Ironically, we had moved into one of the few locations in the country with access to a specialist perinatal mental health service.* The community team attached to Melbury Lodge covered my postcode, and I could have taken my postnatal PTSD to them except for the fact that I was *too* postnatal: the cut-off was one year. This rankled a little. Arthur needed me more than ever. There had been a time when, so long as his bum was dry and his tummy was full, he didn't much mind who was with him, but now Mummy – or 'Muh-yay' as he pronounced me – was front and centre. In many ways, I felt more like half of a dyad than I ever had before.

But rules are rules, and for whatever reason the personality disorder service was also off limits. The only place the GP could or would send me was the local community mental health service. He said, 'It'll be a long wait, I'm afraid.'

———

Emily Dickinson wrote that hope is the thing with feathers. I never understood what she meant by that, unless it's that we must throw a tea towel over its cage if we're ever to get any sleep. The biblical king Solomon wrote, from atop a mountain of gold and wives, that hope deferred

---

* Thanks to tireless campaigning by the Maternal Mental Health Alliance and others, specialist perinatal mental healthcare is now more widely available, although progress is uneven and there is still a postcode lottery.

makes the heart sick. That I could understand. To hope was becoming too disruptive, too much of a risk.

Despair might be the depression that Winston Churchill described as a black dog stalking him. Elizabeth Wurtzel, author of *Prozac Nation*, called it a black wave. I knew what they were getting at. You sense when it's coming after you, even if you don't dare admit it. You run. You keep busy. You go out, meet people, stay positive. You tell yourself that it'll all be fine. Nothing a rest won't sort out. But eventually the dog always pounces, the wave always swamps you. The light fades and fades.

I was overwhelmed. There was unpacking to do, all the new house admin, my Ph.D. thesis ... Writing up research was like wading through a swamp – endless, reeking of the fear that I would never finish. Arthur was suffering with night-time reflux and bellyache, and I seemed to be perpetually arguing with GPs and health visitors that something needed doing beyond pouring endless Gaviscon down his throat. I thought he might have some dietary intolerance, as he was slow to move on to solid food, and the more he ate, the less we slept, but I didn't dare start cutting out whole food groups without any idea of what I was doing.

I have often wondered how much of the too-muchness resided within me and how much was the world around me. How much I was overwhelmed and how much I was overwhelming. It smacked of failure. When I was stretched so thin, I felt like I was failing at everything at once. Most of all, I felt that I was failing Arthur.

The house was narrow and airless, its only windows right at the front and right at the back. I found myself throwing them open and sticking my head out to gulp in the cold. My thoughts were beginning to muddle. Everything was a problem, every obstacle insurmountable, all of it hopeless. Jon was visibly sick of me. Misery, like beach sand, got into everything and chafed, grainy between my teeth. I kept bursting into tears at the post office, supermarket, toddler group ... I'd shout at people before I realised what I was doing.

Perhaps I was depressed, I thought. Perhaps I was bipolar after all. There was no way of knowing, and it hardly seemed to matter any more. I resolved to take one day, one hour at a time. I would do the bare minimum in all respects except where Arthur was concerned, and even there he could spend the odd day in pyjamas, watching people open boxes on YouTube. I thought I could bear it, taking the days hour by hour, if I knew that a day would come when I wouldn't feel like this any more. I told myself over and over that the feeling was temporary. The problem was that the relief was also temporary, and so to self-soothe I fantasised endlessly about killing myself. It was a comfort to know that there was a way out even if I was choosing not to take it.

I was open to a *Wizard of Oz*-style resolution: that moment when Dorothy realises that she's always had the power to go back to Kansas, the trope 'the answer was with you all along'. Although, frankly, if that were the case, I was going to need a few more hints. When I was younger, the doctors and nurses were always telling me I had 'insight'. In fact, I was tripping over insights, new insights every bloody hour, but they never seemed to get me anywhere. Maybe what I needed was to unlock the ultimate insight. If only I could stumble across a wise old woman in a forest, like in a story. 'I can't live like this,' I would tell her.

'It hurts too much.' She would know exactly what I needed to do.

I searched online and found a post on the Netmums web forum in which a psychotherapist had advertised free therapy slots for mothers with postnatal depression. I emailed her, describing my own situation as 'postnatal depression and associated difficulties' – this, I assured myself, was not *un*truthful – and she kindly agreed to see me. The only problem was that she lived miles away, in the countryside north of Winchester. After one bus, one train, two chilly hours at the wrong bus stop, and the best part of £20 spent on a taxi, I entered Olivia's huge, rambling house and felt those feathery flutters of hope unsettling me all over again.

Perhaps this was finally it. The beginning of my recovery. Olivia stated, rather bluntly, that I was looking for someone to rescue me and hoping that she would be the one to do it. I couldn't deny there was some truth in this. I'd prefer to be taught how to rescue myself, but maybe it amounted to the same thing. Olivia also said that at some point I would feel that she wasn't rescuing me fast enough, and then I would rage at her. 'And then,' she concluded, 'work can begin.'

I was afraid that whatever I attempted was doomed, but I knew looking that fear in the eyes was the surest and quickest route to a locked ward. And so I jumped into psychotherapy with both feet – almost literally, as it was a trek over fields and down twisting country lanes from the nearest bus stop, when I found it. I stomped happily enough in all weathers, dosed up with hayfever medicine and playing loud music in my headphones. The journey alone consumed half a week's childcare and intensified pressure to get the Ph.D. thesis done. But it was worth it if I could only, finally connect with someone who understood. I might yet find that I wasn't too lost within myself for another human being to reach me.

If anything, my stint in psychotherapy only confirmed the fear that I was beyond help. The expanse of terrain between what went on in my head and what came out of my mouth was mirrored in the distance between me and Olivia in that room. We spoke about this and that and the other and never really got anywhere. I'd make the journey and finally sit down and all I could think was, I'm exhausted. It wasn't even the travelling. As everything dragged on, as Arthur slept more and more fitfully, as Jon and I had less and less to say to one another, as the thesis became more and more pressing, I had nothing spare, nothing left to give – not even to myself.

—

I've lived enough of my life in survival mode to know how to make a home there. Even when struggle is the main theme, there are illuminated moments, scenes that crystallise in a tableau of perfect happiness that is fleeting but not fake. Those moments, like stained glass, cast coloured light on the stone and dust. I wasn't wholly wretched because there was still Arthur.

I'm certain that, had there not been Arthur, we'd have seen a repeat of my cameo in *One Flew Over the Cuckoo's Nest*, although I don't know what the mental health wards are like in Southampton. There's a decent chance I'd have finally made the grand exit I'd been planning on and off for fifteen years. That I was able to cling on, with bloodied fingernails, to life and to some sort of sanity was not because I was trying harder than before. It was that somehow, without my ever noticing, I had become capable of more. The ability to absorb suffering isn't a virtue but, nonetheless, I could take more of a battering now that I was shielding Arthur.

At eighteen months, Arthur was pure discovery. Every photo was a blur of colour as he dashed on to the next thing. He was averaging at least one new word a day, sometimes three or four, and even starting to put words together. One night, I brought him downstairs and sat him on the sofa while I made a bottle to soothe him back to sleep. He noticed April curled up beside him, meowed at her, stroked her very gently, and said, 'Hello, cat!' Her wearied expression was one of the funniest things I've ever seen.

I bought Arthur a pair of high-top boots, as recommended by the physiotherapist. Our health visitor in Surrey had referred him because he was late with his physical milestones: he crawled, finally, at thirteen months, and could scuttle on all fours at an astonishing speed, but otherwise he was still sitting on his bum. Those green boots were magic. He would sit in his little chair and then raise himself up, with only the slightest support on the back of his calves. It was odd to see him upright. He looked older. He circled the periphery of every room, fingertips against the walls, like someone on an ice rink for the first time. He would be walking soon.

I read once that we don't have any memories before the age of four. Arthur wouldn't remember those days, the days of me and him. He wouldn't remember the crises that seemed so momentous as they were happening, like the time when he absolutely did not want to get off the

Postman Pat ride in the shopping precinct. A queue was forming, and I had to wrestle him into the pushchair, his little body rigid and resisting. He wouldn't remember how no amount of sympathy or explaining or firmness could help. I do remember.

I remember wishing I could tell him, when he was all red-faced and flaily-fisted, so frustrated that I wouldn't let him do everything 'by self' and make all his own decisions, that one day he'll be an adult and then he can play in the sink all he likes. And I remember his lottery-winner face when I came in from the kitchen with a plate of cheese and crackers for his lunch, how he would hurry to sit down. I remember the breeze through his golden hair as I pushed him down the high street. The curls at the nape of his neck. The fire engine that passed and how we both pointed and nee-nawed at it.

I remember how we swept the gravel off the garden path together. I held the end of the broom, he held the middle, and we both said *whoosh* as we cleared the path. I remember him on the sofa, watching *Peppa Pig*, as I got him into pyjamas and kissed his still-tiny toes. Those memories, even the stressful ones, are stars in a dark sky. They aren't sullied or soured because I was so unhappy so much of the time. In fact, they're all the sweeter because they were wrenched out of suffering. I kept my notebooks, and I wrote everything down, so that in my worst moments I could coax the memories back and hold them close.

—

One day, I arrived home with Arthur and a narrow manila envelope was waiting on the doormat. I ran over it with the pushchair as we came into the hall, so that it was crossed with a damp streak. As I picked it up, my name was half visible, pushed above the top of the crinkled plastic window. Somehow, I knew that this envelope contained details of an assessment appointment from the community mental health service. I felt it. It felt like a clenched fist inside my chest, unfurling fingers, a familiar tightening around my throat.

The letter might be something else so long as I didn't open it. I wavered. I could remove myself from this whole process, and I would be free from the worry and disappointment for ever. But that also meant giving up. It meant accepting that I would always be this way and feel this way. And what of Arthur, who was more awake and more aware with every day that passed? He saw me cry sometimes. He heard me argue with his dad. I was deluded if I thought I could contain this ache and struggle within myself, if I thought I could continue to sob my heart out through nap times and cut myself on the sly, and Arthur would never know or be affected. I had to persevere, for his sake if not my own.

The assessment was in two months' time. I looked up the address online and saw a photo of a glass-fronted building set into a cluster of streets to the east of the city centre. I'd never been there, or anywhere closer to it than the marina about half a mile away. The journey was daunting enough. It would mean finding the right bus, inevitably getting lost on the way . . . all so that I could sit in front of a stranger and fail to communicate anything. How could I tell them what it was like? How being me is so unlike being them? All the things that have happened? There would be oceans between us – there always were – and I would be outwardly composed and inwardly crumbling to bits.

That seemed to get worse as the years went by. I was so afraid of medical professionals – or, more accurately, of patienthood – that I was compelled to gear up for every interaction as if it were a job interview, to ensure there wasn't a single chink in my armour, not a scrap of vulnerability left. I was sick of these encounters, the false intimacy that felt more like a one-night stand than anything else. Sick of churning out, on demand, the sort of things you might only disclose to a close friend late in the evening after too many pints. The things that keep you awake at night. My words, so well chosen, hung in the air amid the posters peeling off the walls, the half-closed blinds, the clipboard, and, behind that, another name I wouldn't remember, another indifferent face.

I went to the appointment. It was over almost before it began, with the unanticipated outcome that the referral was rejected. I was not mad enough, or else I was the wrong sort of mad, and so I was discharged back to the GP. Was there nothing else for me? I asked the nurse who did the assessment. He said that if I thought trauma was my problem, I could contact a rape crisis service. He handed me a leaflet, which I stuffed into my rucksack and never looked at again. As he tapped the keyboard for the final time, I pinged back through cyberspace to the GP's desk.

I wandered, lost, through unfamiliar backstreets. It was grey and overcast that day, a restless wind disturbing the litter on the pavement and the sea rumbling away just out of earshot. There was nothing to do but go home. As I scanned timetables at bus stops, I thought how strange it was to be simply turned away. My teenage years had been an endless series of appointments I didn't want to go to, and wouldn't have gone to, had it been my choice. When did I start leading this dance?

It all began with the discovery of my self-harm. That moment in the locker room when time stopped and shuddered, like a film paused on an old television set, and the eyes of twenty girls were on me. My secret, exposed for all to see. Everyone was shocked. My parents were distraught. The doctor was concerned. The headmistress was disgusted. I was deeply ashamed. And yet I couldn't stop hurting myself.

Since then, I had swallowed every tablet, listened to every theory, tried every self-help technique, and I still couldn't stop because I needed it to cope with being me. Once I was an adult, self-harm was easier to hide, and easier to ignore. I was allowed to get on with it, which was what part of me had wanted all along. Yet another part of me clearly did not want that because here I was, taking buses to the city centre of my own free will to tell mental health nurses about it. Somewhere, my thirteen-year-old self was scoffing at this.

The habit was woven into me as the scars were woven into my skin. I couldn't remember how it felt to live in a body unmarked. But what had changed in the last year or so – and this was only just beginning to dawn on me but must have been all too evident to the mental health nurse who did the assessment – was that I wasn't in any danger. I would never again attempt to end my life. I had always been loved, but now I was needed. I belonged to someone. Although there was always a whisper, urging, '*Go a little bit deeper, cut like you really mean it*' – that voice stepped into the ring against my love for Arthur and it lost every time.

Still, I wanted to believe I was worth helping even if I wasn't in mortal peril. I wanted to believe that my experience of being alive was something that mattered. That everyone's experience of being alive is something that matters. It was never about the self-harm, not to me. It was about why I needed to self-harm in the first place. It was about the suffering that, after all these years and all these diagnoses, I still didn't have a name for or a means to communicate.

Just like that, the system which had held me for so many years dropped away. It left a space in which slowly, gradually, painfully, something else would begin to emerge. Recovery, that blurred shape on the distant horizon, was a mirage. It always had been. No one was pretending any more that it was possible. To recover means to get something back; how could I get back what I never had? I have never been like everyone else. I have always felt too deeply, hurt too deeply. I have always found most people alien and inscrutable. I've never felt at home here. There was nothing to recover. I could only begin to forge something new.

It wasn't a revelation, or even a conscious thought. There was no cartoon lightbulb above my head. It just happened. It happened as invisibly and organically as a foetus developing in the womb, or a girl becoming a woman, a process undetectable until already half complete. Plants are growing long before they break the soil. You just don't know it when all you can see is a heap of dirt.

I wonder if you, reading this, have ever felt that same despair. I think of you all the time as I'm typing away, and often as I'm not. I wonder who you are, and why you picked up this book in the first place. I wonder if you've ever felt that you can't live like this. That you've tried everything, and nothing helps. That doors have slammed in your face, or they've opened and led you nowhere. That you're desperate, and you're out of ideas. I've nothing to offer that doesn't sound trite, but I'll offer it anyway. There's always potential for something to shift, for the unknown to come knocking. It's never too late for everything to change. Maybe for you, as for me, it's already changing, and you just can't see it yet.

I don't mean that it was right that I was turned away. Neglect was not the saving of me. It was dangerous, even. It meant managing all my crises in-house, and there were dicey moments and close calls. And I was caring for a toddler, struggling to shield him from it all. It wasn't right. I should have had what I needed: care that was actually caring, and relevant to what I was going through. Surely we can do better, as a society, than to offer something that's often worse than nothing, and offer that to only a few?

When I walked out of my last-ever mental health appointment, I had no idea that things had already started changing for the better. I just thought I was fucked.

Birthday Cake

*Surviving is not a state in which one gets beyond death;
instead death remains in the experience of survival and life is
reshaped in light of death – not in light of its finality but its
persistence.*

Shelly Rambo, *Spirit and Trauma:
A Theology of Remaining*[1]

Winter and spring 2016

As Arthur's second birthday approached, I was flooded
by the same accelerating feeling of doom as the year
before – the same except that it was worse. It started ten
days ahead of the birthday itself. Arthur slept through that
night, a rarity – we were still struggling with reflux – but
I dreamed I'd left him in a crèche, having travelled to collect some award of which I was completely undeserving. I
returned and found the windows dark, the doors locked,
and no answer to my banging and yelling. I broke in. That
was a lengthy process, increasingly panicked, and made no
sense at all. It involved a high tower and bizarrely, at one
point, a helicopter.

When I eventually got into the room, it was dim and loud and squalid, full of babies and toddlers, no adults in sight. I scanned the children – *not mine, not mine* – then spotted the back of Arthur's head. Someone had placed him in a corner, facing the wall, in just his vest. I rushed to him and scooped him up. He was soaking wet, and I was wet, face down in a pillow damp with tears and sweat. Half awake, I staggered across the landing to his bedroom.

There he was, or rather, the shape of him in the dark room. He was sprawled on his belly, nose to nose with Chewy Bear. I put my hand on his back and felt the familiar rise and fall. Then I went to the bathroom to sponge the dream and the panic off myself, but it clung like an invisible film over my skin.

Two days later, I was on the number seventeen bus trundling down the high street. Arthur was at my mum's. I wasn't thinking about anything much, just watching the familiar succession of shops pass by, when suddenly there was a stabbing pain in the back of my left hand. I looked down and there was a cannula in my hand. The tube was about a half an inch in diameter, the point at which it crossed into and through my skin obscured by white tape. A narrower, flexible tube passed out of the cannula and trailed down the aisle of the bus.

I was on the bus and there was cannula in my hand. It hadn't been there before, but it was there now. I could see it and feel it. My hand was swollen and bruised. Carefully, I moved my fingers up and down. I looked to each of the other passengers in turn. No one was behaving as if anything were amiss. I swallowed hard, a great lump like a pebble in my throat. My mouth was parched, my breathing shallow. Not knowing what to do, I did nothing.

The cannula was there for about ten minutes, as the bus crawled through traffic, then I blinked and it was gone. It returned that evening, only for a few seconds as I was settling Arthur off to sleep. Then a few times after that, I felt the same sudden throb but, when I looked at my hand, it seemed completely normal.

The ghost cannula, I reasoned, must be a memory out of place, or out of time. When had there been a cannula? There was one when I was readmitted to hospital, when Arthur was a few weeks old. I didn't think it was that one. When else? Something hovered, like a dream half-remembered in the morning. Something about a slow, painful shower and trying not to get my hand wet. That was all I had.

Soon after, I watched a documentary following two women at Melbury Lodge. It was an odd decision, to have chosen to watch it then of all the days in the year, but these annual PTSD comeback tours always awakened a drive to investigate. What had happened, exactly? What couldn't I remember? If I could ascertain the facts, if I could solve the puzzle, perhaps these ghosts of events would be appeased and finally lay themselves to rest. The previous year I had searched online to find out how to see your own maternity notes. I put in a subject-access request to the hospital, parted with £50, and received a vast and largely unintelligible stack of papers in the post. This year I would watch the documentary, scanning rooms I'd been in like a detective reviewing CCTV.

On the battered leather sofa that had followed us from home to home, and with our dinner in bowls on our laps, Jon and I watched our 2014 play out on the television. The surroundings were as familiar as if they belonged to me, but the mothers inhabiting them were total strangers – like a film of someone else living my life, or like I'd been uprooted, and another woman planted in my place. One of the two mums, Hannah, slept in what had been my bedroom. And there was Dr Gregoire, just as I remembered him. Sometimes he talked to Hannah or to Jenny as he had talked to me, and sometimes he spoke directly to camera. He said: 'Physical illnesses can cause suffering in some cases, so terrible cancers can cause people to be distressed and in pain, but mental illnesses *are* suffering. They are at the very root of where suffering lies, which is of course in our heads, in our brains ...'

That was what I used to say, right at the start when I first got hauled up for self-harming at thirteen, only explained far more clearly than I ever could have. At times I had wept with frustration because I couldn't articulate what my problem was, because the problem was pain, and nobody wanted to hear that.

Since then, I had come to view myself as they viewed me, as a complex case, but really, it was overwhelmingly simple. Not the symptoms – those were ever-shifting, overlapping, indistinct, because they were simply the manifestations of pain, or my responses to it. They were never the point. Eradicating them was never the point, not really. The symptoms – the behaviours, if you like – they were what happened when suffering exceeded my capacity to withstand it. Yet I did withstand it, by any means necessary. As I was shunted around, referred from this doctor to that, from this service to that, I was running in circles, holding up my pain to anyone who would listen, telling them, '*It hurts. Please believe me. It hurts too much, and I can't bear it. Please show me how to make it stop.*'

Watching the mother and baby unit on screen, I felt an extraordinary tug, a wrench not unlike what I felt in the edges of my scar when I stood up too quickly or turned myself at the wrong angle, except that it wasn't quite pain. It felt magnetic, drawing me back, again and again, to the birth and everything after. If my life were a route mapped out, that was where X marked the spot. Something was hidden there, something I was searching for.

I thought of my own conversations with Dr Gregoire, and how he had seemed to know all about me at first meeting, even things I hadn't told anyone. 'Trauma re-awakens trauma,' he said. I thought about the complex PTSD diagnosis, and the instinctive gut rightness of it, and the discomfort of framing as trauma-ridden my comparatively cosy childhood, and how I carried that ambivalence, and then how it had all been eclipsed when I left the mother and baby unit and was diagnosed with borderline personality disorder.

I began to doubt that I had a personality disorder. In fact, I began to doubt that anyone has a personality disorder. The more I learned about personality disorder, not as an objective scientific reality but as a construct, the more it seemed, as Dr Gregoire had said, to be a nonsensical way of understanding people's problems, and also a rather nasty one. It was invented by a German psychiatrist in the 1930s, and termed 'borderline' because patients were believed to be on the border between psychosis and neurosis. More recently, the name was deemed confusing and stigmatising and so it was changed – at least, in some instances – to 'emotionally unstable personality disorder'. I have some bad news for whoever came up with that name: it's not any better.

For me, personality disorder was a character assassination that, once bestowed, was confirmed by anything I said or did, whatever I said or did. A narrative violence that was insidious, different from the physical violence of being pinned to the floor and injected with sedatives, but no less traumatising. It held a megaphone to the lies that trauma was already hissing in my ear, and it shattered my confidence to parent.

When I stopped identifying as personality-disordered, it was a liberation, and it brought me back, hesitantly, to complex PTSD. Since leaving the mother and baby unit, I'd realised that Nan's death had affected me more than I was able to accommodate at the time, and of course a lot had gone on since. Much of my trauma was inflicted by the very people who were supposed to be helping. But in a way, that was irrelevant.

Most of all, I realised that trauma shouldn't be defined by the event. It should be defined by the effect that it has. That PTSD and complex PTSD aren't mental illnesses: they're mental injuries. If you get a physical trauma, say something whacks you over the head and you turn up at A & E, they aren't going to assess that injury according to whether it was a brick or a spade that hit you. They're more likely to look at how much your head is bleeding.

Most of us experience potentially traumatic events over the course of our lives: bereavement, assault, bullying, divorce … Shit happens, and none of us are exempt. Whether or not we're traumatised depends on a complicated range of factors: our genetics, our age at the time, and how we're supported or, indeed, not supported, to name only a few. Two people can have an identical experience and one will walk away relatively psychologically intact while the other is left in pieces.[2] Many people with PTSD and complex PTSD, even those who have lived through the most shocking atrocities, will tell you that someone else has had it worse. It's the shame talking. It's saying, 'I don't matter.' What doesn't matter is whether what's happened to you is better or worse than what's happened to someone else. It's not a competition, certainly not a competition you'd want to win.

If I was slow to cotton on to this, it's poor consolation that the medical community seems slower still. Complex PTSD was added to the International Classification of Diseases (ICD) in 2018, meaning it's become a recognised condition that health professionals can diagnose and, at least in theory, treat.* It's defined as: '*a disorder that may develop following exposure to an event or series of events of an extremely threatening or horrific nature, most commonly prolonged or repetitive events from which escape is difficult or impossible (e.g., torture, slavery, genocide campaigns, prolonged domestic violence, repeated childhood sexual or physical abuse)*.'[3]

To me, this seems backwards, both in the sense that it's unenlightened and, more literally, placing the cart before the horse. It discounts all manner of things: the loss of a parent in childhood, for example, or childhood neglect, or trauma inflicted by systems of oppression like racism or homophobia . . . that is, unless incidents are deemed suitably dramatic. There's an unpleasantly voyeuristic, peanut-crunching feel to it, this relentless focus on *what happened to you*. I wonder when we will stop demanding

---

* The eleventh revision of the ICD was released in 2018 and endorsed by the World Health Organization in 2019 but didn't officially come into effect until 1 January 2022.

that people hold up their worst memories and ask, 'Does this count?'

There was truth in what Dr Gregoire said to me at the mother and baby unit, even if I wasn't ready to hear it at the time. I think most people would have found my birth experience traumatic, to some degree, but it was compounded by everything that had gone before. Traumatic events aren't isolated; they happen in the context of a whole life narrative. Of course, that's not to say that trauma was at the root of every difficulty I'd ever had. Complex PTSD wasn't the whole picture, and perhaps I would never know the whole picture, but I was beginning to think that might be all right.

———

I didn't plan a birthday party for Arthur that year. Instead I invited his grandparents and uncles and aunts to pop in to see him and have cake, staggered so they wouldn't all be there at once. I was trying to be kind to myself, in my torn, ambivalent way. I decided to buy a little play kitchen, as much for myself as for Arthur, and shopping for it was a pleasure. Miniature wooden pots and pans. A teapot and milk jug. Salt and pepper shakers. A chef's hat. I wrapped them all in bright paper.

The night before Arthur's birthday, Jon and I stayed up late assembling the cake that was my most ambitious culinary effort so far: an engine constructed out of a chocolate swiss roll with Jammie Dodgers for wheels, and a Tunnock's teacake topped with a Rolo on the front. It was all held together with toothpicks. More swiss roll cut in half formed the carriages of a train and was piled with sweets. Chocolate fingers for a railway line. It was extravagant, needlessly so.

Fuck it, I thought, surrounded by half-empty bags of confectionery, as I arranged a plastic Peppa Pig to be picnicking with her family as the train passed. I was tempted to have Peppa tied to the tracks with liquorice shoelaces while a moustachioed villain – Bertie Bassett? – cackled nearby. Arthur was unlikely to appreciate the joke, so I lifted Peppa's arm to wave to the train instead. I was surprised to note that I was enjoying myself.

I don't mean to suggest that an acute worsening of mental health symptoms is solved by baking cakes, any more than by tea or baths or whatever else is currently in vogue for fobbing off the desperate. But birthday cakes did become my favoured method of managing the impact of birthdays on my post-traumatic stress. They affirm Arthur's rightful place in the centre of things – Arthur as he is now, not as a jaundiced infant – and for me, they're the right combination of hands-on creativity and logistical problems to solve. That's not to say I don't wind myself up in the process of making them. I absolutely do, and Arthur is banned from the kitchen partly so as not to spoil the surprise, but also partly because my language gets increasingly unsuitable for little ears.

The cake-making is sweetened by memories of my own childhood birthdays. My Auntie Viv was (and is) a cake genius, and she produced some absolute triumphs. There was a cottage with Shreddies for roof tiles, a duck with a pink handbag, and, best of all, a Sindy doll inserted into a huge dress made of cake. Even as a little girl, I noticed the love and care that went into my birthday cakes. I wanted Arthur to have that. That was why I started taking custom requests.

There was *Hey Duggee* for his third birthday, Super

Mario for his fourth, *Splatoon 2* (emphatically *not Splatoon 1*) for his fifth. Then it started to get interesting.

A few weeks before he turned six, Arthur said, 'I'd like a cake of the Elder Dragon, which is a *Minecraft* dragon I've just made up. He lives in the End and he's friends with the Ender Dragon and he wears a crown.' I borrowed a plastic crown from Nick's daughter's Barbie doll.

The seventh birthday cake was *Minecraft*-themed again, a series of characters arranged on top of a grass block. I'd neglected to account for the fact that these blocks are cube-shaped, as tall as they are wide, and I had to take out all the shelves in the fridge to make space for the icing to set. When asked for his verdict, Arthur said, 'You did as good a job as it's possible to do with your skill level.'

The following year, he requested, 'A cake of Darth Vader's head, actually shaped like it.' He mimed the shape of the helmet with his hands to indicate that the head should be three-dimensional. 'And when you bring it out, instead of "Happy Birthday", I want everyone to sing "The Imperial March".' I did – just about – manage to make a Darth Vader-head cake, and we sang 'The Imperial March'. Which is also quite a funny soundtrack to the annual revival of my PTSD.

Birthdays do keep coming. After the second was harder than the first, I was terrified that the trend would continue. Wasn't time supposed to be a healer? What if it just got worse and worse each year? By the time Arthur was out for his first pint I'd be . . . Well, I didn't know what I'd be. But after the first few birthdays, they did become slowly, although not steadily, less invasive. There was still that tidal force pulling me back, but I was more able to wade through it without being knocked off my feet.

I don't know what people mean when they talk about 'resolving' trauma. You can't exorcise it, like a malevolent spirit, or erase it. I'm not sure that you can even end the chapter, close the book, neatly tie up the loose ends that dangle all over the place and stray into everything. If you can, that must be the work of a lifetime. Perhaps others, more magnanimous than I, have learned to embrace something so prickly and monstrous, to accept the unacceptable, but I haven't. I think it's shit. Trauma is what remains, and you have to learn to make space for it. Then, as time passes, it's still there but you've grown around it. I've heard the process of grieving described as concentric circles: as you grow, there's more room, and so you bump up against your grief more gently and less often. I think trauma is like that too.

As I write this, we're eight birthdays in. I'm still learning to accommodate the emotional hangovers and general fragility that comes with them. I still remind myself that it's understandable to find it a tricky time, that it doesn't mean I don't adore and celebrate Arthur, and that it's not making his day all about me. The scar across my pelvis bristles and stings. My phone assaults me with a photo of myself, grey and swollen and dead behind the eyes, a tiny orange baby held up to my chest. But there's no hallucinating any more. As the years pass, the terror-stricken feeling is morphing into something more like grief – grief where what was meets what could or should have been – and even a sort of thankfulness.

Having been close to death in a hospital bed, and now upright and busy and swearing in my kitchen, I can't help but be impressed by the resilience of my body. Survival isn't defeating death, as if we'd been engaged in a fistfight. For me, survival is remaining in this body and being altered, carrying death with me in these physical and mental scars all the days of my life. It's acknowledging the suffering that doesn't go away, but nonetheless being here, not consigned to the past but invited to the present. I am thankful to be here.

Lived Experience

Liberation is always in part a storytelling process: breaking stories, breaking silences, making new stories. A free person tells her own story. A valued person lives in a society in which her story has a place.

Rebecca Solnit, 'A Short History of Silence'[1]

Autumn 2016

I was bloody well going to finish that Ph.D., more out of stubbornness than anything else. Any hopes I might once have cherished for an academic career had dwindled to nothing. I had no teaching experience. I wasn't willing to move around the country from university town to university town every year for as long as it took to land a permanent post. I couldn't give myself over to the whole project as I might have done before Arthur was born. I didn't want it badly enough. I was twenty-eight and had no idea what I planned to do with my life, except that I knew that I did plan to be alive. And I planned to be Arthur's mum. The rest I would have to figure out as I went along.

Arthur had been referred to a gastroenterologist at our

local hospital, finally, after his reflux and general collywobbles worsened so that he was demonstrably losing weight. We were trying out medicine and dietary changes to help, but it was slow progress. I kept a diary of everything he ate and then his symptoms overnight. I dreaded those broken nights. Arthur had transitioned from the cot to a floor-bed, and more often than not, I slept sprawled between floor-bed and floor.

In hindsight, it seems miraculous that while only sleeping in twenty- or forty-minute bursts, I was upright and at least semi-coherent, never mind finishing a doctorate. After a bad night, the world would shimmer like a mirage. Tears were permanently prickling at my eyelids. Jon and I continued to circle the marital drain. Somehow, I managed to hold it together, just about. Arthur needed me, and I was still so afraid of traumatising him by falling apart.

I hurled myself at my thesis. It was the first time in years that I'd embraced a topic wholly outside myself and allowed that topic to consume and transport me. Surely that's what it means to be 'into' something – to be inside it, submerged, carried along, blurring and blending so that you're part of it and it's part of you. To forget yourself in the experience, and then to find yourself in it. I was constructing a collective biography of about ninety women who had taken chastity vows in the ninety years between about 1450 and 1540. I got to know them, as far as you can get to know people who died half a millennium before you were born, and I wrote 90,000 words about their lives and why they matter. The process was complicated and bewildering and sort of maddening; there were times when I despaired over finding a way through, but it was such a privilege to be able to do it, and to be funded and paid for it.

One afternoon, I was alone in the house, alternating mouthfuls of strong coffee and chocolate hobnob while getting acquainted with my latest library haul. Among the volumes was *Original Letters, Illustrative of English History*, compiled by some dusty antiquarian in the early nineteenth century. I'd never been that interested in History with a capital H – the History of kings and battles and parliaments. The History of men having tedious arguments. Men in iron helmets, men in powdered wigs, men in top hats, all waving their dicks around over the centuries. It seemed far removed from the past that I wanted to know about. I had only borrowed the book because it contained a transcript of the earliest surviving letter to Henry VII from his mother, Margaret Beaufort. (You might remember her from an earlier chapter: she was the one bawling her way through the coronation, which must have put something of a dampener on proceedings.) That letter begins: '*My own sweet and most dear King, and all my worldly joy . . .*'

All my worldly joy. I whispered the phrase to myself, and saw Arthur running into soft play, wildly performing the Makaton sign language for 'friend' that he'd learned off CBeebies, as if the action itself were enough to cause new friends to flock to him. It was perfect. Margaret Beaufort was only thirteen when she gave birth, recently widowed amid the violence of the Wars of the Roses and sheltering at the home of her brother-in-law. The labour was lengthy and difficult, and neither she nor the baby were expected to survive. She never had another child. Instead, she devoted herself to putting Henry on the throne – and that's why we had the Tudors. Later she became a vowess, founded two Cambridge colleges, and was an artistic and literary patron and a scholar in her own right.

People often asked me why I chose to study vowesses. It wasn't their religion that appealed to me, or the celibacy, or even the proto-feminist angle. What defined vowesses was that they were liminal, on the border between laypeople and professed religious, like monks and nuns. They inhabited a space halfway between the convent and the world. I don't mean that literally in terms of where they lived: vowesses lived wherever they liked. That's the point. To become a vowess was to continue one life while embarking upon another. Each woman navigated that dual life in her own way.

I've always felt out of place, like I didn't fit in. I love my working-class family and I loved my middle-class education, but at home I was too posh, and at school I was too common. Then, after some confusing feelings about girls, and about boys, I realised that I'm bisexual. Too gay to be straight and too straight to be gay. I had no idea what to do with that. And there was something deeper, underneath it all: an unbelonging that wasn't about social class or sexuality or anything I could put my finger on ... I thought that university would be where I found myself, a self that was clear-cut and acceptable to people around me. But when I got there, I was dismayed to discover that I was still me. I was still the person who said, 'Well, actually it's complicated ...' and was met with baffled politeness.

If I couldn't be fully in one camp or another, I was excluded from both. At least, that's how it had felt. Historians had described vowesses that way too. Almost nothing had been written about them, aside from a smattering of articles in the mid-1990s, one of which speculated that the reason no one had heard of a vowess was because their vow excluded them from studies of laypeople and yet neither did they qualify for convent studies.[1] Where vowesses were mentioned, usually in passing, they were portrayed as obscure, reclusive figures. That's bizarre, really, because vowing was commonplace among well-to-do widows in the later Middle Ages. The profession itself was widely acknowledged, and vowesses were active not just in religious circles but across public life. The vocation was a marginal one, but these women were not marginalised.

As I spent more time with my vowesses, I was struck by their freedom. They owned property and lived where they chose. They were as involved in religious life as they wished to be, and they integrated into wider society as much or as little as they wanted as well. As such, their lives looked completely different from one another's. Some were young mothers, busy with small children, and others were old ladies widowed in their last few months of life. Some were noblewomen running vast estates, and others were merchants' widows running their husbands' businesses. Some lived in convents. Some founded schools. Some were leading ladies in their parishes. Far from being isolated, they were embedded in all these different communities – in monasteries, in parish churches, in towns, in their families. They simply chose their own places to belong.

Vowesses taught me that liminality is a position of strength. 'You don't have to be one thing or another,' these long-dead women seemed to call to me, an echo scarcely perceptible, muted by centuries. Then, a little crazy with caffeine, I'd read a phrase like *all my worldly joy*, and for a moment their voices were startlingly clear. 'You can be both. Be a hundred things at once if you like. Have your cake and eat it – after all, it would be a shame to have cake and not eat it.'

Medieval religious life was varied and vibrant and ambiguous, and I decided that I want my life to be those things too. If other people are confused, ultimately that's their problem. I can only expend so much energy explaining myself. There are people, rare jewels, who grasp this multiplicity of self immediately and instinctively. They're usually the ones who also have a dozen overlapping identities and interests, and witness first-hand how everything colours and enhances everything else. I've learned to hang on to those people.

When Arthur was born, I travelled to the limits of my body, and then a bit beyond. After that experience of birth-in-death and death-in-birth, life and death could never again be opposites, or even separate. The past invaded the present. Death invaded life. The boundaries could never be what they were, and I had to learn to make a home in the space between. I was well placed to do that after a quarter of a century on the margins and fringes of things. Trauma, like most things that are shit, has unexpected benefits, and mine nudged me into claiming my status as edgeperson – with a little help from my dead friends.

As we began to get more sleep, I could expand my own diet beyond the two food groups of sugar and caffeine and relinquish that fierce focus on getting through each day. I could hold a conversation again, take an interest in other people. I could enjoy Arthur as well as love and protect him. All these abilities sleep deprivation had stolen without my ever really noticing. They returned, too, by stealth. I don't remember realising that I could, once again, complete a thought, or that I could pounce upon ideas as they scurried across my consciousness. But my thesis notes, those vast documents of half-sentences, arranged themselves into something like coherence. I began to see an end in sight.

Three months later, I boarded a train and sped through the countryside, back to the university town where I'd lived for almost ten years. As I turned to climb the hill, I noted which buildings had changed and which were the same. A restaurant had closed. Some of the shops and cafés had new names. I was surprised by this, stupidly, as if I expected the town to freeze whenever I wasn't in it. I waved to the Cardboard House across the petrol station forecourt, but it didn't acknowledge me. The town felt deserted, despite cars rushing by. Further up, I passed the turning for the cottage that housed the first months of my pregnancy. Beyond it was the pub. I might venture into the village, I thought, pass more of my old haunts, but I didn't like the way it was all the same yet different. There was something eerie about it. And anyway, I had a thesis to submit.

On a campus full of strangers, I handed in two bound and laminated copies, and then I did go to the pub. I met Julie and her partner there, even though they'd started to prefer another pub in the village, and no one else, because our other pub friends had all moved away. Hayley had gone to Yorkshire, where I liked to imagine her in a flat cap, surrounded by whippets. I drank rum and Coke for the first time in a couple of years, and that, too, was the same but not the same.

I woke up the next morning in Julie's spare room,

hungover and with an unpleasant taste in my mouth, like coins retrieved out of soil. I was glad to have visited, and it was lovely to see Julie and Pete again, but I was beginning to realise that the girl, or young woman, I was when I lived in that town was dead, and that I wouldn't go back for anything.

—

As I was finishing my thesis, I found myself integrated into a small but flourishing online perinatal mental health community. It had started with the mums I befriended soon after Arthur was born, and evolved into a wider network of parents, doctors, midwives, and the like. People had been running their own initiatives for decades, dotted all over the country, and those dots were connecting into a bigger picture. A movement was building. It wasn't so much about raising awareness, although that was part of it. We wanted to improve the care and support that was available. Most of the country still had no specialist perinatal mental health provision at all.

My blog and Twitter account were busier than ever before, and I began to receive a steady stream of emails and messages: acquaintances, friends of friends, fellow historians, even total strangers would contact me to pour out their grief around their birth experiences. I'd never meant for that to happen, and it was a little overwhelming, but I was thankful to be trusted with something so private and so raw. For the first time, I felt knitted into a wider fabric of humanity, and I was awed by the weight of the suffering that so many other mothers were silently hauling about. It wasn't just me, nor just a dozen of my friends online. What a revelation to discover that birth trauma was so common and so hidden.

I had been asked to comment on drafts of a 'perinatal mental health toolkit'. This was a collection of resources for GPs, developed so that they would be better equipped to recognise perinatal mental health problems and arrange the right support at the right time. I'd emailed back and forth with the doctors working on this toolkit, and they had invited me to the launch in London over the summer. I went along, and during the Q & A, I asked some typically forthright questions about how mothers who had lived through these experiences would continue to be involved in the work of improving perinatal mental healthcare. My view was – and still is – that academic knowledge and clinical experience have their place, but you could spend decades in a library or consulting room, and you still wouldn't understand what this shit feels like unless you'd lived it. What's needed is for different perspectives, different kinds of expertise, to come together. It's like a jigsaw puzzle for which we're all carrying different pieces.

My question was answered by a woman in a beautiful dress, brightly coloured and scattered with butterflies. Maria worked for the Maternal Mental Health Alliance (MMHA) on 'Everyone's Business' – a campaign for specialist perinatal mental healthcare to be available to every family, regardless of postcode. She said they were keen for mums with 'lived experience' to join their supporters so they could invite us to collaborate in their work. I followed this up by email the moment I got home and through the front door.

Maria emailed again about six weeks later and asked me to give a talk at an event. The aim was to bring together people who could really make a difference to the quality of local services, so that they could learn together, share ideas and solutions, and ultimately make things better. Would I take a thirty-minute slot, including questions? Yes, I replied immediately. I would absolutely do that. Maria's colleague phoned and talked me through it all, making sure I was comfortable to share my own experiences. There were seven of these events planned, and I could take my pick. I signed myself up for the very first one. The topic was: 'The difference it makes to have or to not have a specialist perinatal mental health service.'

I could name a dozen ways in which things might have played out differently, had there been a perinatal mental health service where I lived when Arthur was born. There could have been actual preparation and planning during my pregnancy, mitigations for the high-risk period known to be just over the horizon. Someone could have identified my birth trauma earlier, and intervened before it got so utterly out of hand. Maybe we wouldn't have needed to go into hospital. Even if we had still gone to Melbury Lodge, I wouldn't have been stuck with Annette after I came out again. I might have had therapy for my PTSD so that it didn't return to fuck me over every time Arthur had a birthday. I might have dodged the personality disorder service.

I couldn't change what had happened to me – that was done and consigned to the past – but I might be able to change, or at least influence, what happened to someone else. I handwrote pages of notes about the birth and the tongue-tie, the flashbacks and intrusive thoughts, the bleeding and the trip to A & E, the bus ride to the GP surgery and the doctor's visit to my house, back to A & E with Michael Caine, right up to going into the mother and baby unit ...

This talk, I realised, was far too long. I started over, focusing on the process of seeking help after I realised that something was wrong. I identified and named each instance where a perinatal mental health service could have created a different outcome. Then I practised with the stopwatch on my phone and got the talk down to twenty minutes. Still, a dam had burst. After fifteen years of medical professionals telling me what was what, it was my turn to tell them, and I would find other opportunities.

It was October when I stepped into the morning rush at Paddington, automatically reaching down for a little hand that was at home. The crowd surged, almost lifting me off my feet, but I found and boarded the Hammersmith and City Line. The Tube carriage shrieked and shuddered like a launching rocket as it snaked through the darkness. It made me dizzy – the speed of it, the weight of everything above. I got off at Moorgate. London was scaled up more than usual that day, people creeping and swarming over its surface like reams of ants. I made my way along a row of towering buildings to my destination and was directed up to the eighth floor.

The venue was arranged in a café-style layout, and it struck me immediately that I had made a terrible mistake. People stood around in twos and threes, catching up on the latest news, discussing their journeys, enjoying filter coffee and pastries. Those I'd met before greeted me and smiled and made pleasant chit-chat and I smiled back, my pocket burning all the while with index cards covered in handwritten scrawl about haemorrhages and suicide and whatever else I'd vomited onto them. I'd edited the talk to make it shorter; why hadn't it occurred to me to take out the really awful bits? This was not what the nice people were expecting, I was sure. It could not be what Maria had in mind when she invited me to come and speak. They were going to be absolutely appalled.

And there, with his back to me, sat Dr Gregoire. He was typing at a laptop, working intently on something. I felt like a child who has seen her primary-school class teacher in the supermarket. You always imagined – or at least I did – that at 3.15 p.m. all the teachers went into the supply cupboard and plugged themselves in at the mains until morning. You might concede that they ate food, and even that they shopped for food, but you absolutely did not expect to see them in Tesco on a Saturday afternoon, wearing jeans and buying crisps. If you were ever unlucky enough to witness your teacher dropping a multipack of salt-and-vinegar into their trolley, there was nothing to do but gape and hover nearby. Should you dash off and pretend you hadn't seen them? Should you hide? Should you go over and say hello?

Should I go over and say hello to Dr Gregoire? Should I still call him that, or was he Alain, since I was no longer a patient? What was the etiquette for bumping into one's former psychiatrist some two and a half years later? My brain popped up a frantic series of error messages: *No prior experience. No frame of reference for this interaction. Not recognised.* I found myself backing out of the room. He looked busy anyway. Better not disturb him.

I scurried to the nearest toilet and shut myself in a cubicle. There, I sat on the lid and considered my options.

Attempt to flee? Wouldn't be my proudest moment.

Apologise and say I didn't feel up to giving a talk after all? Awkward, and still letting people down.

Write a new talk, extremely quickly? Difficult. Possible? Probably not.

I spread the index cards across my lap and started scribbling over and around my own words, crossing out the grimmest bits, adding a light-hearted aside here and there. I thought I might be able to do this if I could soften the edges of those splintered weeks, if I could only edit myself into something more palatable.

Inky-fingered, I glanced at my phone.

'*Shit*,' I hissed through my teeth. The event would be starting. I stuffed my belongings into my bag and hurried back, troubled by a gnawing sense of unravelling, of nakedness. Was my dress tucked into my knickers? Was there loo roll stuck to my shoe? Had I forgotten to put shoes on? I hovered at the door, inspecting my clothes, recalling the time I got halfway down the road in my slippers and the time I almost collected Arthur from my mum's with the hoover instead of the pushchair. Externally all seemed present and correct. Internally I was all wrong.

In seconds, I was standing at the front of the room, among flipcharts and Post-it notes, index cards in my trembling hand. A sickening realisation washed over me: the rewrites had rendered my notes illegible. I looked out over thirty or forty expectant faces. Maria smiled encouragingly. There was an awful moment in which all I could hear was my own ragged breath. And then I did what seemed the only thing to do: I gave my talk. The original version. I'd practised so much I had it off by heart.

My voice swept over other sounds: the clink of coffee cups, the murmur of hastily concluding conversations, the scratch of biros on paper. As I reached the episode when I was on the bus with the pram, I noticed those noises had retreated, cleared a circle in which I stood alone. I couldn't recall anyone listening to me that intently, ever. I'd never felt all eyes in a room fixed on me and not wanted to run away and hide. Instead, I felt strangely exultant – powerful, even.

And then it was over. The spell was broken. I fled to my seat too soon, only to be called back so that I could answer questions.

The next coffee break was like being mobbed. Everyone wanted to talk to me intimately, one to one.

'Laura, I just wanted to say . . .'

'I wanted to tell you . . .'

Some spoke of their own experiences of birth and early motherhood. Some described women they supported in their work. Some wanted to pile on praise that was as well-intentioned as it was embarrassing. I was staggered that any of these people gave a shit what I thought, and more so that it was the messy, unfiltered bits of my narrative that seemed to resonate most. I also felt, rather suddenly, that I needed to curl up and go to sleep.

I did speak to Alain, or rather, he came to speak to me. It was surreal, disjointed – him, twinkly-eyed and energetic as ever; the miniature cup and saucer in my hand; conversation in snatches; and people milling around us. I attempted to fill him in on an abridged version of the last two years, while also attempting not to stand in anyone's way, or block access to refreshments, or spill my coffee. He asked if I would consider giving other talks in future.

That was how we started our 'double act' lectures on

complex PTSD. We've trained thousands of people coming to work in new perinatal mental health services.

Later, I would explain to Arthur that I teach people how to help mums with their mental health, and that I tell them about what happened to me when he was a baby.

'You mean they all have to just sit there, while you talk and talk and talk?'

'Yes,' I said. 'Yes, they do.'

Epilogue

*One can only show how one came to hold whatever opinion
one does hold. One can only give one's audience the chance of
drawing their own conclusions as they observe the limitations,
the prejudices, the idiosyncrasies of the speaker.*

Virginia Woolf, *A Room of One's Own*[1]

Summer 2022

Being professionally mad is an odd way to earn a living.
These days I'm something of a Jill of all trades, giving
talks and lectures, sitting on advisory panels for new mental
health projects and services, setting up peer support ... It
turns out that relevant lived experience is an asset in pretty
much any work with the ultimate aim of relieving human
suffering. I like mental health research best of all. Finding
things out and writing them down continues to hit my joy
buttons, and leading focus groups and interviews, I get to
have meaningful conversations without the need for too
much small talk. Big talk is where it's at.

I still research and write about my vowesses and the
world in which they lived. It doesn't pay my rent or even

the bar tab, but I don't see that as a reason to pack it in altogether. Why should I not be half medievalist, half lunatic for hire? At least as much as limitations of time and money will allow. I like that I am forever straddling the border territory between everything and everything else. When I sit around a table with health professionals, I'm halfway between them and their patients. I try to act as a bridge, or a translator. In many ways, a Ph.D. on medieval vowesses was the perfect training for it.

Working in lived experience roles is not without its hazards. I often feel I have to prove myself, to shine very brightly in meetings so that the doctors and academics will revise their initial opinion of me as the 'service user' – someone second-rate, less skilled, only useful for rehearsing my own trauma. They ask me to tell my story, as if I have one story. As if I could select one story, like out of a chocolate box. As if my stories were fixed and not constantly evolving. There's a pressure to represent *lived* experience rather than *living* experience, to be safely recovered, positioned on the correct side of a neat before and after.

Most days I share deeply personal and sensitive information about myself with strangers and near-strangers. I make decisions on the spot about how much detail to offer, when to share and when to hold back, and those judgements vary based on all sorts of factors. I've shared a lot with you over the course of this book, but I haven't told you all my secrets. This is merely a carefully curated selection of my secrets. I'm still terrified about how it will be received, and what future ramifications there may be, not only for myself but possibly for Arthur. I hope I've made wise decisions. Sometimes, in this book and in my work, I feel like I'm walking a tightrope between privacy and disclosure.

At other times, I feel like a magician. Magic has been defined as 'the putting into practice of this: that the subtle rules in the dense'.[1] In other words, what happens invisibly and internally – our thoughts, feelings, griefs, prejudice – tends to dictate what happens visibly and externally, in our behaviour. Our behaviour, individually and collectively, dictates what happens to every one of us, all around the globe. It's a sort of magic to harness one's internal world and use it to influence the external world. My inner landscape has always been a particularly lively place, a private and sometimes lonely place. To offer it, and to see it cross that boundary between me and you, a boundary that once seemed so impenetrable – that is a gift.

At the mother and baby unit, Alain told me that I was a survivor. It felt wildly uncomfortable, as if I were appropriating something that was not mine to claim. I even looked it up in the dictionary – 'A person who survives, especially a person remaining alive after an event in which others have died.'[2] It's true that some of the girls at Maplewood didn't grow up, and that I've lost good friends because they were failed or punished by mental health services. You can say that they lost their lives to mental illness, but the people I knew didn't die because of that, not really. They died because the safety net didn't catch them, because it disintegrated and clung like a spider's web the moment that they fell into it. They died because they asked for help, and someone didn't believe them.

I'll come to the conference and drink the nice coffee and have you reaching for your hankie, but I will never not be angry. I carry with me all those friends and contemporaries who walked the path alongside and didn't make it. I am here, and they are not, and I don't know why, and it isn't fair. The system of mental healthcare that we currently have in place is not fit for purpose. I have to tell you about that because there are so many people who can't.

Now I work with, and sometimes within, that same system to bring about improvements. But I do worry: if I climb too far down, will I be consumed? When do I become an enabler, one of the cogs that keeps this destructive machine whirring? I want to work collaboratively with everyone, whatever their professional background – to win hearts and minds – but half of me will always wonder if I should have come into that room at all. Perhaps I should be marching outside with a placard on which I've printed *BURN IT ALL DOWN*.

I will always be in that room, trying to speak hard truths in a calm voice that will be considered credible. At the same time, I will always be in the streets, screaming the same truths over the roar of indifferent traffic. I try to hold these tensions within myself, and to honour them for what they are. I try never to allow myself to nod along when the humanity is hoovered out of the conversation, and everyone speaks only in acronyms. I try not to let myself drift into spaces that hurt people more than they help. I don't always get it right, but I am learning.

'Someone is coming to help you,' the self-checkout assures me.

I stand stupidly in front of my half-scanned groceries while machines beep and plastic bags rustle and voices swim around me.

After what feels like for ever, a man comes and waves his staff card in front of the scanner.

'Thanks,' I say, but he's already gone.

Trudging home with my groceries, I think about those times when we're promised that someone is coming to help us, and we wait and wait, and they never do. Then we muddle along as well as we can. If we're lucky, we might stumble into our own solutions. I was lucky. When I stopped looking outwards and started looking inwards, I found what I needed after all.

Part of me would like to end this book: *I've solved mental illness. You're welcome.* Wouldn't that be nice? I'd like to say that we lived happily ever after. Even that I've crossed an invisible threshold between well and unwell, and I'm waving at my younger self from the other side. In all honesty, I can't say that – not because it would be a lie, but because that binary isn't how I see things any more. I was never very good at mapping myself onto it in the first place.

I can say that I'm happier than I've ever been, and that life is easier than it ever was. I'm still someone who feels deeply, gets anxious easily, is socially awkward, and tends to be gloomy on occasion. I'm still me. It's just that now I wouldn't be anyone else.

Arthur and I live on a housing estate to the west of Southampton. Jon is just a few minutes' walk away and visits most days. April has reached the grand age of seventeen and is cantankerous as ever. Jane Hunt resumed her rightful place on my bed some years ago. Bethany Fleamarket and One-Legged Margaret are here too, supervising my home workshop in which I repair vintage and antique dolls. I think it's funny that in this healing, which has been slower and deeper than the cure I once anticipated, I have indeed been transformed – but in the opposite direction. I am more myself, not less.

When the voices around me fell silent, I finally heard the stifled murmur of my own voice. I felt stirring all the things I used to know before. I began, slowly and imperceptibly at first, to lean into my instincts and rediscover old channels within myself. I know that sounds vague and abstract, and a bit 'woo' in a pound-shop mysticism sort of way, but that's not what I mean. It comes back to self-care, not hand cream or candles or colouring pencils, but a commitment to working with who I am and not against. I've discovered, and rediscovered, the things that are helpful for me. In doing so, I found ease and pleasure in being who I am.

When everything is painful and overwhelming, my mind offers its own sanctuary in imagination, music, writing, immersive interests, a weird preoccupation with the distant past – and these function as a sort of inbuilt refuge, a bomb shelter at the bottom of the garden for when the world feels too dangerous, or simply too much. I will always be someone who feels things deeply. That's why I came inbuilt with the tools to withstand that. I didn't learn to use those tools. I unlearned not to use them. I had to wade back through the years to the girl I was before anyone took me to the doctor about it, and I had to reclaim her.

Debates rage endlessly about the correct way to approach extreme distress and experiences like voice-hearing or finding oneself inexplicably unable to get out of bed, paralysed by terror or despair. Where do these things come from – mental illness, trauma, some secret third thing? How should we respond? Should someone write a prescription? Or ask, 'What happened to you?' Or normalise it? Everybody seems to have a view.

It puts me in mind of a book I loved when I was a little girl. The book was called *The Lady with the Alligator Purse* and it was about a child who drinks vast quantities of soapy bathwater.* His mother anxiously summons a doctor, a nurse, and, for some reason, a lady with an alligator purse.

'Mumps,' says the doctor.

'Measles,' says the nurse.

'Nonsense,' says the lady with the alligator purse.

'Penicillin,' says the doctor.

'Castor oil,' says the nurse.

'Pizza!' says the lady with the alligator purse.

If there is a right answer, I'm willing to bet it's the answer that feels right for you. It's your distress and it's up to you what sense you make of it – or not. Whether you opt for the penicillin, the castor oil, or the pizza, it should be your choice and we don't all have to come to the same conclusions. But don't wait, as I did, for some so-called expert or authority figure to bestow enlightenment, or to tell you who you are. I wasted so much time asking people directions from places they've never been.

That's not to say you can't consult, of course. Take advice, put out a survey if you like, just don't be fooled into thinking that anyone knows better than you do. And you don't have to be alone. I hope that you find your own

---

* There are multiple versions of this story, all based on an American school-yard rhyme most often known as 'Miss Lucy had a baby ...'

Jemmas and Harriets and Hayleys along the way, because they are what makes it all survivable.

Looking back, I see fifteen-year-old Harriet handing me her copy of *Prozac Nation*. I see Giddy strumming his guitar and writing in my leaving book. I see Nick headed towards the bin on a bicycle stacked with board games. I see my mum sleeping on an inflatable mattress so that she can help me look after my new baby. I see Hayley packing my clothes for Melbury Lodge. I see Esther and Alain Gregoire too, having a normal day at work. If they seem like minor characters in the story, that's my failure in telling it. They were the lanterns on my path. There were others, too – I couldn't name everyone in this book. If you're one of those people, I hope you know how much I love you, and how much I owe you.

And of course, there's Arthur. He's the most wonderful person. I feel fortunate that he's someone I would want to spend my time with even if he weren't my son.

Motherhood is love on steroids. It's sitting on the carpet at 3 a.m. so you can hold hands through the bars of the cot, and it's hiding in the bathroom with a glass of water to chew a replacement Chewy Bear so that it doesn't look new. It's also watching your enormous eight-year-old playing on his Xbox and thinking, God, you are so beautiful. How is it even possible for anyone to be that exquisite? It's lying awake at night because one day something truly awful might happen to him and you might not be able to prevent it, because all the possibilities have taken up permanent residence at the end of your bed, and somehow you must live with them. Becoming a mother has wrecked me and put me back together in a different order. It's the maddest thing I've ever done, and the best.

Postscript

Finishing *All My Worldly Joy* seemed almost impossible. Perhaps a memoir can never be complete, at least while its author is still alive. Not only am I still learning, still evolving, and changing my mind about things every other day, the past will not sit neatly where it's put. Recently I discovered something which lit it all up from a different angle, creating shapes and shades I hadn't seen before.

As you know if you've read this far, I had always thought there must be a reason why I felt different from other people and why I found my ordinary life quite so painful and overwhelming. I thought there must be something wrong with me, and I spent years questing to find out what that something was. Eventually, I decided that although there are certainly things that are unusual about me, there's nothing much wrong. I found ways to embrace the difference and minimise the suffering.

Then, quite unexpectedly, I stumbled across the answer to my original question. I'm autistic.

Throughout my lengthy and eventful career as a psychiatric patient, neither I nor anyone else ever considered autism. Autism meant no social skills. It meant severely disabled. It meant a mathematical genius. It meant an eleven-year-old boy who loves trains. It meant everything, apparently, everything except me.

I had been diagnosed with dyspraxia while at university, after I read about it and asked my support worker to refer me for an assessment. Dyspraxia is a little like dyslexia, except that instead of reading and spelling, it affects my ability to co-ordinate actions and movement. It explained why I'm so clumsy and always lost. It explained why PE was so mortifying, and that one memorable sports' day when I accidentally threw a javelin backwards into a crowd. It was why I had never managed to ride a bicycle or drive a car. I'd assumed all those things were just because I was crap, so an alternative explanation was welcome relief. But I didn't think dyspraxia had anything to do with my mental health.

It was while I was working on *All My Worldly Joy* that I became aware of autism – actual autism, rather than the *Rain Man* stereotype I'd grown up with and never thought to interrogate. This was nothing more intentional on my part than mindless scrolling through social media when I should have been doing something else. I came across the budding online autism acceptance movement, and autistic influencers, tweeters, Instagrammers, TikTokers, and bloggers who share their own experiences. Just like when I first learned about birth trauma, it was not the people who were trained and paid to help who came up with the goods, but those who were suffering themselves.

Some described an overlap between dyspraxia and autism. Huh, I thought. That's interesting. I read up on it. I read about how autistic people often have highly focused

interests, precocious abilities in childhood, unusual sensitiv-
ity to light and sound, social anxiety, a direct communication
style, an intolerance for small talk, a vivid imagination, a
tendency to be perceived as quirky or eccentric and to feel
overwhelmed by their emotions ...

Still, I wasn't inclined to pursue a diagnosis. I had enough
of those. A great stack of them. A cupboardful. I tried to put
it aside, but it nagged at me. *Was* I genuinely autistic? Had
I been autistic all along, and was that the reason my life had
taken the course that it had? Would I ever know for sure?
Here was another potential explanation for a whole bunch
of things, and with it, potential for relief and an antidote to
some of the shame I'd been lugging around all my life.

But diagnoses, I argued with myself, are less an objective scientific reality and more a social construct. They
evolve along with the societies who invent them. They're
often helpful, but not always. And these autistic traits and
characteristics are probably relatable to most people, to
some extent. What if this is personality disorder all over
again? What if it's just confirmation bias?

It's a bit spooky, though, isn't it? came the counter-
argument. Look at this photo of you, in your first term at
school, lining up coloured blocks on the carpet while other
children play together. In this one you're eight, clutching
two enormous dolls in your chubby arms and endeavour-
ing to smile for the camera, but accidentally producing a
facial expression that can only be described as utterly ter-
rifying. Look at the sheer number of hobby-based
spreadsheets you've created over the course of your life.
This one is called 'Sankyo for the Music' and it contains
nearly 1,500 different arrangements of tunes for the 3S
music-box mechanism manufactured by Sankyo from 1985

onwards. You made that for fun. Other people watch television. Let's talk about how you plan every second of your time in meticulous detail, how you've listened to the same songs over and over for decades, and the fact that you've felt chronically misunderstood your entire life.

In the end, I decided to book an autism assessment. It wasn't that I needed to know whether I was autistic or not. I knew. The more I learned about autism, the more certain I was. Nor did I think it would be fraudulent to tell people without inviting someone to pass judgement after meeting me only a handful of times. Many autistic people can't access an assessment for all sorts of reasons and that doesn't make them less autistic. What I really needed to know was this: if I put all the evidence in front of someone with qualifications, what would they say?

But I couldn't face the NHS route of arguing my way onto a years-long waiting list, and private assessments cost thousands of pounds. I was stumped, until someone on Twitter recommended a psychologist-led adult autism practice who were more affordable and did remote assessments over video calls. Most importantly, the website emphasised that they viewed autism as a difference rather than a deficit or a disorder. This meant that they used the official medical criteria to render the diagnosis credible, but in all other respects they took a non-medicalised approach.

After a few months on a waiting list, many questionnaires, and four interviews, a psychologist confirmed that I – thirty-four years old and sitting at my laptop, surrounded by dolls – was undoubtedly, unequivocally autistic.

'Congratulations,' he said. 'You're part of a community of wonderful people.'

He explained that being funnelled into psychiatric services in early adolescence and then diagnosed with everything under the sun was 'a common pipeline' for autistic girls. What autism looks like in women and girls is often different from what it looks like in men and boys. Mental health services are slowly catching up to this, as is society more broadly, but female autism is still chronically under-recognised and under-diagnosed. As a result, autistic girls and women are treated as if they're mentally ill until that becomes a self-fulfilling prophecy.

Still, I don't know that health services or the world at large would have been kinder had I been diagnosed in childhood. We're a long way from a society that affirms and celebrates neurodiversity, and in the 1990s and 2000s, we were further still. As a teenager, I might well have seized upon autism as my entire identity in a way that wasn't good for me. So perhaps it's not a catastrophe that by the time I got my answer, I almost didn't need it any more.

One of the first people to hear my news was Harriet, heavily pregnant with her second child. I sent her a Whats-App message, and she replied, 'I must say, I'm not surprised. I wondered that for you a while ago.'

My mum responded similarly. She works with autistic children at my former primary school. I guess she's been well trained for it, raising me. I know she has regrets, and I feel for her. It's cruel that my autism should be so obvious in hindsight when no one knew enough to spot it at the time.

Some people couldn't spot it even after I told them.

'Really?' they said.'You don't seem autistic.'Whether that's because they don't know what autism is, or because I've learned to 'mask' convincingly in some situations, or both, I don't know. Nor do I particularly care.

What matters to me is that it feels like a lamp lit suddenly in a dark room, as no other diagnosis has except dyspraxia and complex PTSD. It feels liberating and sense-making. It's helped me to understand and accommodate my sensory needs, for example by wearing big sunglasses in the supermarket. It had never occurred to me that I don't have to tolerate those glaring overhead electric lights that are like kebab skewers in my eyeballs. Nor did it occur to me that if I were more comfortable, I might be less likely to spin out emotionally. I look like a bug, but people are going to think I'm odd whether or not I try to convince them otherwise, so I may as well wear sunglasses indoors and swing on the swings in the park because it feels lovely.

As I review my past through my new autism sunglasses, I have more compassion for my younger self. As I view the present, I'm more likely to give my current self permission to be who she is rather than to conform to expectations. I'm more likely to forgive myself when I become intensely anxious over things that I know other people would take in their stride, or when I struggle to communicate. I shouldn't need a diagnosis for any of that, but I can't deny that it helps.

It's been less than a year since my autism diagnosis, and I'm still working out what it means. I think some of the difficulties I had attributed to trauma might better be ascribed to autism, but both are clearly present and so really, who cares? What's important is that I manage those difficulties more skilfully, and more gently, than I used to. I think, too, that leaning into my hobbies and interests – things like vowesses, dolls, journaling, collecting strange objects and arranging them in my home . . . maybe all that was so transformational because I was embracing the autism that I didn't yet know I had.

I'm not going to reduce myself to a checklist, not ever again. I want to hold this diagnosis lightly enough that I can set it down when I need to, and to give myself the freedom to shed it altogether if I outgrow it. I have so much to learn, but I do know this: I wouldn't change who I am for anything. That wasn't always the case, and my autism creates challenges and vulnerabilities, but nothing that can't be managed with care and understanding – and several notebooks, of course, a very specific kind of pen, a decent pair of headphones, dimmable lighting, a cat, a hundred dolls, and a large chocolate cake, please, if one's going.

Notes

Bethany Fleamarket

1 Rumer Godden, *The Dolls' House* (Macmillan Children's Books, 2016).

Morning Has Broken

1 *The Devil's Backbone.* Directed by Guillermo del Toro, performances by Marisa Paredes, Eduardo Noriega, Federico Luppi, Irene Visedo, Fernando Tielve, and Íñigo Garcés. Warner Sogefilms, 2001.

2 *Goodbye, Mr Chips.* Directed by Sam Wood, performances by Robert Donat, Greer Garson, and Terry Kilburn. Metro-Goldwyn-Mayer, 1939.

Body Language

1 Muriel Spark, *The Prime of Miss Jean Brodie* (Macmillan, 1961).

Maplewood

1 Roy Porter (ed.), *The Faber Book of Madness* (Faber & Faber, 1991).

The Genius Disease

1 Bianca Stone, 'Reading a Science Article on the Airplane to JFK' in *Someone Else's Wedding Vows* (Octopus Books and Tin House, 2014).

Rota Fortunae

1 Boethius, *The Consolation of Philosophy*, trans. by V. E. Watts (The Folio Society, 1998).

2 John E. B. Mayor (ed.), *The English Works of John Fisher, Bishop of Rochester* (Trübner, 1876), pp. 305–6. I have modernised the spelling.

Titanium

1 George Eliot, *Middlemarch* (Penguin Classics, 2003).

An Act of Infinite Optimism

1 Gilda Radner, *It's Always Something* (Avon Books, 1989).

Rounding Apace

1 Sylvia Plath, 'Metaphors' in *Collected Poems* (Faber & Faber, 1981).

Failure to Progress

1 H. P. Lovecraft, *The Call of Cthulhu* (Norton, 2022).

The Mother-Creature

1 Helena Fox, *How It Feels to Float* (Dial Books, 2019).

When the Bough Breaks

1 Liz Berry, 'The Republic of Motherhood' in *The Republic of Motherhood* (Chatto & Windus, 2018).

2 *The Italian Job*. Directed by Peter Collinson, performances by Michael Caine, Noël Coward, Benny Hill, Raf Vallone,

Tony Beckley, Rossano Brazzi, and Maggie Blye. Oakhurst Productions, 1969.

Melbury Lodge
1 Polly Clark, 'Dora' in *KISS* (Bloodaxe Books, 2000).

Homecoming
1 Lulu Allison, *Salt Lick* (Unbound, 2021).

A Pink Toothbrush
1 Terry Pratchett, *Reaper Man* (Corgi Books, 1992).

Pernicious Motivations
1 Adolph Stern, 'Psychoanalytic Investigation of and Therapy in the Border Line Group of Neuroses', *The Psychoanalytic Quarterly*, 7:4 (1938), pp. 467–89.
2 John G. Gunderson, 'Borderline personality disorder: ontogeny of a diagnosis', *American Journal of Psychiatry*, 166:5 (2009), pp. 530–9. These two quotations were extracted by Rachel Rowan Olive for her one-day training course: 'I is for Insult: Questioning Borderline Personality Disorder'.
3 International Statistical Classification of Diseases and Related Health Problems, Tenth Revision (ICD-10) – F60.3, Emotionally unstable personality disorder. EUPD is the newer name for BPD.
4 *DSM-IV: Diagnostic and Statistical Manual of Mental Disorders*, Borderline personality disorder.
5 The report is dated 2011 and is still available online at the time of publication. See https://www.rcpsych.ac.uk/docs/default-source/improving-care/better-mh-policy/college-reports/college-report-cr164.pdf?sfvrsn=794 16179_2.

That Time May Find Its Sound Again

1 Weldon Kees, 'Small Prayer' in *Collected Poems* (Faber & Faber, 1993).

Mother City

1 Laura Varnam, 'A New Woman at Beowulf's Funeral Pyre' in *The Mechanics' Institute Review* online, 6 July 2022.

Birthday Cake

1 Shelly Rambo, *Spirit and Trauma: A Theology of Remaining* (Westminster John Knox Press, 2010).
2 Babette Rothschild has explained and illustrated this in more depth: *The Body Remembers: The Psychophysiology of Trauma and Trauma Treatment* (Norton, 2000).
3 International Statistical Classification of Diseases and Related Health Problems, 11th Revision (ICD-11) – 6B41, Complex post-traumatic stress disorder.

Lived Experience

1 Rebecca Solnit, 'A Short History of Silence' in *The Mother of All Questions: Further Feminisms* (Granta, 2017).
2 Patricia Cullum, 'Vowesses and Veiled Widows: Medieval Female Piety in the Province of York', *Northern History*, 32 (1996): pp. 21–41 (p. 21).

Epilogue

1 Virginia Woolf, *A Room of One's Own* (Penguin, 2020).
2 Jessica Dore, quoting *Meditations on the Tarot* in *Tarot for Change* (Hay House, 2021), p. 39.
3 Google's English Dictionary, provided by Oxford Languages.

Acknowledgements

Firstly, *All My Worldly Joy* would not exist without Andy Charman, who supported me through the process of writing it. His extraordinary generosity in reading countless drafts, encouraging me, championing me and allowing me to enthuse and rant and wail at him every single week has been something else, and thanks is not a big enough word. I've gained not only a published book, but a very dear friend.

Thank you to Fiona Lensvelt, whose kindness and enthusiasm got the book off the ground; Imogen Denny, who transformed a manuscript into a book with such professionalism and who has been very patient with me; Rachael Kerr, who provided a developmental edit that felt more like a lovely cuddle and still made the book better; and Kate Quarry, whose meticulous attention to detail has spared the reader my numerous mistakes.

Thank you also to Will Atkinson, Anna Simpson, Dan Hiscocks and all the team at Wilton Square, who rescued *All My Worldly Joy* after its former publisher, Unbound (later Boundless), went into liquidation just a few weeks before the scheduled publication date. They have been kind, reassuring and capable in the aftermath of a distressing situation, and I don't know what I'd have done without them.

Mark Ecob designed the cover. We had never met, or even corresponded, and yet somehow, he knew what I was thinking better than I did.

Julie Aherne believed in *All My Worldly Joy* before anyone else. Emily Beecher and Laura Varnam read very early drafts and helped me to figure out how on earth I was going to write this thing. Nick Lowe has lost many hours of his life to listening to my monologues about the themes and anecdotes within the book, along with the minutiae of my life in general. He will never get that time back.

Leo O'Kelly is responsible for introducing me to Weldon Kees. Any dystopian villanelles that may have crept into these pages are entirely his fault.

Thank you to everyone who gave me permission to quote from their work, especially Lulu Allison, Laura Varnam and Polly Clark. Thanks also to Polly for her generous encouragement, which began with our correspondence when she was Poet in Residence at the *Southern Daily Echo* and I was twelve.

Jessica Dore's online newsletter and her book, *Tarot for Change*, have been sources of inspiration and influence throughout, as I followed up on her recommended reading. I've benefitted enormously from attending Rachel Rowan Olive's superb one-day training course: 'I is for Insult: Questioning Borderline Personality Disorder' and from Rachel's art, tweets and blog posts, as well as from online conversations with Heather Cobb, and from the wisdom and solidarity of the mad activist community more widely.

I'm grateful to every single person who supported

the Unbound crowdfunding campaign. Thank you for your faith in me and for your patience. You've been the invisible cheering crowd when I felt like giving up. Thanks especially to all those who helped to spread the word and to those who sent messages of encouragement. Your support has been incredible.

My best thanks and love to friends and family who trusted me to write about them: Jemma, Giddy, Harriet, Mr and Mrs Ramsay, Nick, Hayley, Lisa, Julie, Sarah, Tom, Alain, Maria, Auntie Pat, my brother Tom and, of course, Jon, and my lovely mum and dad. Uncle Graham has since passed away but is lovingly remembered in these pages. I'd also like to thank the great supporters of this book and of my life who have so far escaped mention: Paul Alborough, Jennie Allen, Nikki Clark, Rob Haynes, Ollie Meyer and Emma Nicholson, Diana and Luke Saunders, Lorna Taylor, and Alex and Liz Vintleman.

Last but certainly not least, thank you to Arthur for allowing me to write about our story. I've made some educated guesses about what you might or might not want to be public twenty years from now, so I hope I've got it right, or at least not too wrong. This book is as much yours as it is mine, and one day I hope you'll feel proud of it as I am proud of you.

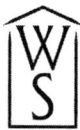

Publication of this book was originally crowdfunded by the author in collaboration with Unbound, before the publisher went into liquidation in 2025. Everyone who pledged their support is listed below.

Wilton Square Books is proud to publish *All My Worldly Joy* and pleased to acknowledge the support of all those who originally made it possible.

Kate Abbott
Abi Adam
Martha Adam-Bushell
Claire Adams
Karen Adams
Stephanie Addison
Julie Aherne
Nisba Ahmed
Lauren Aitken
Rowena Alberga
Kate Aldersey
Jennifer Allen
Rachel Allender
James Alsop
Elaine Amoah
Josie Anderson
Tamzin Anderson
Ariel Anderssen
Lisa Archibald
Kelly Asagba
Mandy Astbury
Debbie Atanasio

Sabra Attrill
Sylvia Austen
Nadia Ayoub
Jemma Bachelor
Sarah Ball
Sakina Ballard
Sasha Barber
Kirsten Barnicot
Tracey Barratt
Caroline Barron
Sue Barsby
Caroline Bate
Alison Baum
Maria Bavetta
Catherine Beard
Helen Bedford
Sheila Beesley
Sabina Begum
Paul Bentley
Giles Berrisford
Amy Bianchi
Elizabeth Biggs

Catrin Billam-evans
Hannah Bissett
Lesley Black
Celia Blay
Helen Bloomfield
Katie Bogart
Alex Bollen
Kirsty Bolton
Charlotte Bonsey
Catherine Boorer
Hilary Booth
Laura Bottini-Porsolt
Amy Bottomley
Casey Bottono
Kathryn Bradley
Lydia Bradley
Jeff Bray
Jo Bray
Sadie Brazier
Dawn Brenchley
Stephanie Bretherton
Shara Brink
Sarah Brown
Brian Browne
Andrew Bull
Kathryn Bundle
Rachel Bunting
Jennifer Burgess
Laura Burgin
Roxanne Burrows
Anna Burry
Hollie Burton
Marcus Butcher
Ashleigh Butler
Ruth Butterworth
Wren Cage
Katie Cairns
Pamela Carson
Hazel Carter
Nicola Carter

Leanne Cartwright
Alexandra Cassie
Emma Catteau
Mary Cava
Barbara Chaitoff
Fiona Challacombe
Samantha Chaney
Debbie Chant
Andy Charman
Rebecca Chilvers
Heather Chisem
Angela Clark
Laura Clark
Nikki Clark
Sue Clark
Rachel Clarke
Sarah Clement
Susan Cleverley
Miriam Coad
Fiona Cobain
Heather Cobb
Allison Colchester-Long
Jonathan Cole
Rachel Colley
Claudia Conway
Sarah COOK
Anne Cooke
Jen Cooke
Heather Copete
Hannah Copley
Helen Cordery
Emma Couch
Elizabeth Coulter
Paul Court
Donna Cowan
Tamsyn Crane
David Crepaz-Keay
Rachael Crosbie
Helen Cross
Katherine Katherine Cross

Erika Cule
Poppy Cullen
Kimm Curran
Ashley Curry
Clare Curtis
Chris Cusack
Emma Custance
Zoe Darwin
Helen Davies
Megan Davies
Lizzie Davison
Fineke Francina de Jong
Lydia Dean
Anna Demarcy
Karen Dempsey
Becky Derham
Sarah Dickens
Angela Dickson
Chelsey Dinneen
Julie Dixon
Joanne Docherty
Clare Dolman
Miriam Donaghy, CEO
    MumsAid
Dan Douglas
James Downs
Jane Drewett
Emma Ducklin
Keith Dudleston
Ionae Duff-Turner
Emily Duncan
Jennie Dunn
Liz Durrant
Vicky Earll
Stef Eastoe
Jo Edge
Amanda Eglite
Chloe Ellis
Linda Emmett
Katy Evans

Dominic Everett
Victoria Fallon
Danielle Fantis
Melanie Farman
Clare Faulkner
Rebecca Fish
Jill Fisher
Maggie Fisher
Jessica Fitzsimmons
Red Fletcher
Vicky Fobel
Sue Forber
Jean Forbes
Valerie Forrester
Jane Foster
Lucas Fothergill
Vicky Fox
Anna France-Williams
Jacky Francis
Charlie Francis-Pape
Ellie Frankish
Jane Franklin
Ruth Franklin
Amy Jefford Franks
Patsy Friend
Miranda Frost
Andi Fugard
Catherine Gale
Katie Gallagher-Cox
G.E. Gallas
Charlotte Gauthier
Anna Gee
Clare Gendy
Lynn Genevieve
Dion Georgiou
Jane Gibbons
Stephanie Giorgio
Susy Giullari
Ben Glass
Hilary Goodman

Pat Goodman
Maggie Gordon-Walker
Rita E. Gould
Su Goulding
Natalie Goult
Emma Grae
Claire Grant
Kathryn Grant
Catherine Gray
Christa Gray
Kenneth Gray
Emily Grayson
Catherine Green
Louise Griew
Eamonn Griffin
Hayley Grocock
Smile Group
Katherine Guyatt
Mark Guyers
Gary H
Rachel Hagger-Holt
Nicola Haggett
Jane Haines
Emylia Hall
Raf Hamaizia
Cleo Hanaway-Oakley
A Hankin
Jane Hanley
Agnes Hann
Laura Hans
Liz Hanson
Elaine Hanzak
Amy Harrington
Emma Harrington
Mark Harris
Wil Harris
Akiko Hart
Sophie Harwood
Kayt Hawkins
Claire Hayes

Sarah Hayes
Emma Haynes
Rob Haynes
Stu Haynes
Laura Helen
Emma Henley
Lauren Herd
Kat Hewlett
Layla Hibbs
Annie Hickox
Sarah Hislam
Sally Hogg
Hayley Holmes
Libby Holroyd
Anna Hope
Janey Hopkins
Hannah Horne
Rebecca Horne
Karen Horstead-Sayer
Stephen Hosking
Stephanie Hovland
Leanne Howlett
Samei Huda
Francesca Hufton
Elizabeth Hunt
Natasha Hunt
Cheryl Hunter
Allan Isdale
Rebecca Ison
Maria Ivanov
Elizabeth Jane
Sarah Jane
Jane Jefferies
Sian Jenkins
Jill Jensen
Sommer Johansen
Taryn Jolliffe
Hannah Jones
Lauren Jones
Sarah Jones

Katarina Jonsson
Mira Kafantaris
Nina Kaler
Joan Kavanagh
Laura Keable
Sophie Kennard-Holden
Jo Kennedy
Danielle Kershaw
Matthew Kilburn
Emma Jayne Kilford
Shona Kinsella
Teresa Valdez Klein
Charlotte Knapp
Lisa knowles
Tanja Kovacic
Helene Kreysa
Carrie Ladd
Mireille Lam
Beckie Lang
Annabel Laughton
Pete Lawrence
Ewan Lawrie
Melissa Lee-Patrick
Kev & Liz Lendon
Fiona Lensvelt
Lucy Lenton
Shareen Lewin
Judith Liddell-King
Ashley Long
Jessica Long
Lucy Long
Fiona Lovell
Nick Lowe
Irene lowry
Jacqueline Lynas
Jo MacDonald
Aki MacFarlane
Philippa Machin
Helen MacIntosh
Samantha Maddocks

Meabh Maguire
Rosie Mallen
Hannah Marsh
Imogen Marsh
Michelle Mason
Johanna Mason-Laurence
Stef Maudsley
Anna May
Shelley McBride
Katrina McChesney
Katherine McDonald
Julia McGinley
Maddie McMahon
Sara McMahon
Sarah McMullen
Ashley McNally
Aidan McQuade
Julie-Anne Meadows
D Mellars
Celia Mill
Michelle Miller
Heather Milne
Amy Milton
Eleanor Molloy
Linda Monckton
Mary Monro
Coffee Monster
Becca Moore
Ashley Morgan
Lynette morgan
Lisa Morriss
Alasdair Morton
Pippa Moss
Rachel Moss
Kelly Moulds
Kasia Mullan
Yu Müller
Patricia Murphy
Lorraine Murray
Maggie Murray

SJ Murray
Carlo Navato
Lorna New
Scott Newby
Maisie Nicholls
Emma Nicholson
Sue Nicholson
MS NIMH
Miranda Noble
Liz Nolan
Abigail Norman
Alison Norman
Zoe Norris
Elisha Nunhofer
Natalie Nuttall
Rachel O'Brien
Leo O'Kelly
Mark O'Neill
Maryann O'Connor
Rachel Rowan Olive
Kate Olver
Sally Osborn
Bob Packer
Ruth Paginton
Gwen Papp
Rachael Parker
Maggie Parry-Mantel
Graham Partridge
Darren Paskell
Jenny Patterson
James & Sue Pavey
Alison Pedley
Russell Perera
Jayne Persian
Benjamin Peters
Gill Phillips
Lena Phillips
Charlotte & David
   Pignon
Teresa Pilgrim

Esme Podmore
Rebecca Pope
Ruth Prentice
Candyce Prevett
Jo Price
Liam Pywell
Gwen Rahardja
Lisa Ramsey
Rachel Ravey
Claire Reece
Anita Reed
Isy Reed
Hannah Reeve
Ruth Revell
Sofia Reynolds
Catherine Rice
Tom Richmond
Jacqueline Riddles
Janet Riggs
Lorelei Rivers
Ellie Mackin Roberts
Rachel Roberts
Denise Rogers
Melanie Rogers
Kinga Rona-Gabnai
Jane Rose
Sitar Rose
Philippa Ross
Catherine Roy
Harry Rutherford
Nat Rutherford
Naomi Salisbury
Christoph Sander
Felicity Sankey
Louise Santhanam
David Santiuste
Diana and Luke Saunders
Kate Saunders
Jess Savage
Kavita Savjani

Richard Sawrey
Charlotte Schindler
Sharon Scotford-Smith
Jane Ariztegieta Scott
Sarah E Seaton
Laura Seebohm
Becky Selbie
Debbie Sells
Shirley Shailer
Kirsty Sharrock
Susannah Shaw
Dani Shearing
Helen Shearing
Nicola Sheldon
Helen Sheppard
Sian Hardy Shevlin
Sonia Shuter
Martina Di Simplicio
Neil Simpson
Irene Smith
Jan Smith
Michelle Smith
Hannah Snashall
Eamon Somers
Madeline Spicer-Barrett
Molly Spokes
Rose Stanford
Stavros Stavrou
Alison Stephenson
Jackie Stevens
Ellen Stewart
Rebecca Stokes
Eleanor Sturdy
Angela Style
Lucy Sullivan
Nicola Summers
Celia Suppiah
Emma Svanberg
Nikki Syvret

Toshie Takata and Stuart
    MacFarlane
Ingrid Tamuyeye
Kerry Taylor
Lorna Taylor
Scotty L Taylor
Alex Templeman
Julian Templeman
The Frank Curtis Library
Jack Thomas
Clare Thompson
Ruth Thorne
Claire Thornley
Alex Thornton
Sarah Toler
Tom Tora
Siobhan Towsey
Heather Trickey
Amy Tubb
Jo Tucker
Lesley Turner
Sophia Ufton
Saskia Vanpeene
Laura Varnam
Mark Vent
Nadine Verstraten
Bryony Vickers
Maria Viner
Liz Vinton
Ruth Vorstman
Ruth Waghorne
Tom Wainwright
Joanne Walkeden
Charlotte Walker
Melita Walker
Jenny Walsh
Megan Walsh
Emma Ward
Miranda Ward
Henna-Sisko Warner

Ruth Waterton
Ursula Watkins
Jay Watts
Andy Way
Gemma Webb
Hannah Webb
Sara Webb-Kröhl
Juliana Wekel
Elizabeth Welch
Alex Westcott
Verity Westgate
Suki Westmore
Brian Wharton
Helen Whelan
Suzanne White
Bethany Whiteside
Valerie Whitlow
Denise Wiesner
Jen Wight
Flo Wilcock
Marie Wilkinson
Harriet Williams

Myfanwy Williams
Ruth Williams
Mark Willis
Katy Willmont
Naomi Wills
Hannah Wilson
Sally Wilson
Jon Wood
Moira Wood
Steven Wood
Tim Wood
Tom Woodman
Angela Woods
Sylvia Woolley
Michelle Wright
Sheryl Wynne
Richeldis Yhap
Emily Young
Kathryn Young
Sue Young
Hisham Ziauddeen

A Note on the Author

Laura Richmond is a researcher, campaigner and consultant who works to improve mental health care, especially for parents and families. She was admitted to a psychiatric mother and baby unit after the birth of her son in 2014. After completing her PhD in medieval history, she switched careers to use her own lived experiences of complex trauma and autism in partnership with charities, universities and the NHS. *All My Worldly Joy* is her first book.

A Note on the Type

The text of this book is set in Bembo. Created by Mono-type in 1928-1929, Bembo is a member of the old style of serif fonts that date back to 1465. Its regular, roman style is based on a design cut around 1495 by Francesco Griffo for Venetian printer Aldus Manutius, sometimes generi-cally called the "Aldine roman". Bembo is named for Manutius's first publication with it, a small 1496 book by the poet and cleric Pietro Bembo. The italic is based on work by Giovanni Antonio Tagliente, a calligrapher who worked as a printer in the 1520s, after the time of Manu-tius and Griffo.

Monotype created Bembo during a period of renewed interest in the printing of the Italian Renaissance. It con-tinues to enjoy popularity as an attractive, legible book typeface.